Y0-CUN-582

A Woman's Health

Gillian Strube

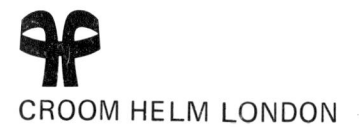

CROOM HELM LONDON

© 1980 Gillian Strube
Croom Helm Ltd, 2-10 St John's Road, London SW11

British Library Cataloguing in Publication Data

Strube, G
   A woman's health.
   1. Women – Health and hygiene.
   I. Title
   613'.04244   RA778

ISBN 0-85664-940-6
ISBN 0-7099-0411-8 (pbk)

Printed and bound in Great Britain by
Redwood Burn Limited
Trowbridge & Esher

CONTENTS

Introduction	9
1. A Woman's Health	12
2. The Role of the Primary Health Care Team	25
3. Menstruation	35
4. Love and Sex	46
5. Conception and Contraception	60
6. Pregnancy, Birth and Post-natal Care	70
7. Marriage	83
8. Family Life	93
9. Middle Age	106
10. Old Age	114
11. Depression and Anxiety	129
12. Women Alone and Handicapped Women	140
13. Team Support for a Woman's Health	152
Index	162

INTRODUCTION

A Woman's Health and the Primary Health Care Team

A woman's health has always been a nebulous concept, a fragile and incomprehensible quality easily destroyed by hysteria, venery or vapours. For centuries, bizarre, crude and often lethal procedures were performed on women to drive out demons or cleanse them of *furor uterinus*: the excessive sexuality held responsible for everything from amenorrhoea to uterine cancer. Myth and ritual surrounds the subject.[1] Modern medicine enables us to explain many of the conditions which the ancients found so mystifying but it is not at all clear that we are any nearer than they were to understanding the health of women in our own society. In theory, technical advances should have resulted in universally high standards of health. The reason that this has not happened is as deeply shrouded in mystery as were the causes of disease to earlier generations.

Symptoms of ill health in twentieth-century Western women are commonly attributed to neurosis and treated with tranquillisers, a practice as ineffective and only slightly less cruel than the excesses of the past. Lack of comprehension of the health of women characterises medical practice now as it always has.

Health services are often accused, with some justification, of providing a sickness service when they should be providing a health service. Resources are spent on trying to pick up the pieces when illness and disability are established instead of concentrating on improving the health of the nation and preventing disease. This is expensive and inefficient and results in unnecessary suffering. However brilliant the surgeon, or sophisticated the medicines, no one is ever as well after treatment as he would have been if the condition had never occurred. It also has to be admitted that the majority of disease is virtually unaffected by medical treatment, which often does more harm than good, or is merely palliative.[2]

These arguments are not new. They have never carried much weight or affected health policy because not only is it patently obvious that disease must be treated and the sick cared for but also everyone is only too well aware that he will one day himself be a patient, suffer an illness and need, or at least want, medical care. There is also an almost mystical belief that, as well as ensuring that he will be successfully treated if he develops a disease, supporting the system in some way protects the individual from becoming ill. Many smokers have a regular chest X-ray, more than half believing that it protects them from developing lung cancer.

Few people would support the contention that all our resources should be spent on prevention. A service for the sick is necessary and should be as good as it can be. It is equally clear that there should be greater emphasis on health as a positive individual attribute and on the prevention of disease and disability.

Women are the largest consumers of health services. This is partly because they are, by tradition, in charge of family health and sickness and therefore seek, receive and interpret health care on behalf of children and the elderly. It is also due to the fact that women suffer from ill health to a greater extent than do men. The reasons for this are complex and ill understood but social and domestic factors are certainly as important as biological ones in determining the incidence of their 'dis-ease', in its most literal sense, and have to be taken fully into account in both the maintenance of health and the management of illness.

It is clear that if the health of women is to be improved it must first be better understood. To do this it must be examined in its overall social context.

Those working in primary care are in daily contact with women in all states of health and sickness. They are in an ideal position from which to observe and to learn about the health of women and then to try to improve it.

Many individual general practitioners, health visitors and district nurses have been committed to this work for years but the more the health of women is studied, the clearer it becomes that the traditional format of primary care is inadequate. Health has its roots in all aspects of a woman's life and many and varied skills are needed to preserve, improve or restore it. These cannot be provided by any one person or even by a number of individuals working separately. A woman's backache cannot be treated without considering her marital difficulties nor her antenatal care properly conducted without help for her housing problems or knowledge of her other children. To be fully effective, all the individuals involved must work closely together.

This is generally recognised and few general practitioners now work in isolation from colleagues in other related disciplines. They are grouped together with health visitors, community nurses, midwives, ancillary staff and others to form primary health care teams.

Introduction

However, the setting up of these teams of itself gives no indication as to how they should work and what they should be trying to achieve.

The natural tendency is for each member of the team to continue to work separately, in relative isolation from his colleagues. The health visitor sees the young children and their mothers, the community nurse tends the sick, the midwife the pregnant women. There is no obvious and immediately pressing need to change. This is especially true of the doctor whose training and previous methods of practice have habituated him to taking decisions alone, without discussion, explanation or justification. A radical change of attitude is needed in him if he is to work as a member of a team.

Determination, vision, flexibility, tolerance and a great deal of hard work are needed from everyone if teamwork is to succeed. When it does succeed, the achievement of each member is enhanced.

I will discuss in detail how primary health care teams may be made to work in the last chapter.

The health of women is central to the health, happiness and prosperity of the whole nation both now and in the future. The primary health care team promises to be the best method yet of advancing it.

This book is an attempt to identify some of the foundations of the health of women and to examine ways in which the resources of the health service, in the form of primary health care teams, can be used to increase understanding of it and to raise its standard. It is written with the British system in mind but the same principles apply to other highly developed countries.

Notes

1. H. Graham, *Eternal Eve* (Heinemann, London, 1950).
2. I. Illich, *Medical Nemesis* (Calder and Boyars, London, 1975); T. McKeown, *The Role of Medicine* (Nuffield Provincial Hospitals Trust, 1976); P. Rhodes, *The Value of Medicine* (Allen and Unwin, London, 1976); J.S. Bradshaw, *Doctors on Trial* (Wildwood House, London, 1978).

1 A WOMAN'S HEALTH

What is Health?

The World Health Organisation definition of health is: 'Health is a state of complete physical, mental and social well-being and not merely the absence of disease or infirmity.'

If this is taken literally, it is abnormal to be absolutely healthy. Everyone experiences symptoms of one sort or another from time to time. Headache, backache, indigestion, anxiety and many others are common. The incidence of such symptoms and their severity varies from one person to another. Those with the highest incidence also seem to have the greatest frequency of disease or what might be called a low health quotient. Those with the lowest incidence of symptoms and of disease have a high health quotient. The rest of the population lies between these two extremes forming a spectrum of healthiness.

The health quotient of an individual is not fixed and unalterable throughout life. It changes from time to time and is influenced by a number of factors. Just as the performance of a child with a given intelligence quotient, and even the intelligence quotient itself, can be improved by skilled teaching, the health of people with a low health quotient can be improved by appropriate help and the health quotient raised.

The precise form this help should take and how best it should be provided is not yet clear and forms the basis of much discussion.

The Health of a Woman and her Family

Some of the women on every doctor's list attend the surgery very seldom, usually those with a high health quotient. Others come again and again (low health quotient). The differences between the two groups are not immediately obvious. It is not a question of age, social class, poverty, parity or the ages of their children. One woman with a large family of young children seems to get by without seeing a doctor for months or years on end, while another, apparently similar, is in every week. It is not that one family neglects important symptoms or that the other comes unnecessarily, although this is a factor. The frequent attender really does have more episodes of illness, her children really do have otitis media more often than the children of the other woman. The health quotient of the whole family is low. In addition to clinically diagnosable illnesses, the sickly family suffers to a greater extent from undiagnosable illness. This does not mean that it is imaginary or neurotic. The child really is ill with pallor, anorexia, perhaps a fever; the woman really does have menorrhagia or crippling backache but the doctor can find no medically recognisable cause for it. This mother is also unable to cope with minor illness in the family without medical help. Apart from the misery their ill health causes for themselves, the worst of these families give rise to enormous problems for the doctor and the rest of the health team. They take up a great deal of time and cause much irritation. They often have to be fitted in as extras in an already fully booked surgery because of the potentially serious significance of their symptoms. These same symptoms — combinations like headache and vomiting, or abdominal pain and anorexia, mean that the doctor must take every episode seriously and exclude important organic disease which might need urgent treatment. At the same time he knows that it is unlikely that on this occasion, out of many, the woman has an ectopic pregnancy or the child meningitis. He is irritated, anxious and, at the same time, feels guilty. He is annoyed at 'wasting time' and 'getting behind'. He feels that he has failed in not making an accurate diagnosis. If he invents one to satisfy the patient, he feels guilty. If he tells her he does not know what is wrong, he is a disappointment to her and she looks more anxious. If the doctor cannot help her, who can? She expects treatment, or he feels she does, even if he cannot give her a diagnosis and he finds himself prescribing inappropriately. It is all he can do. The sickly child receives a course of antibiotics; the bleeding woman, hormones, or a tranquilliser, or both. The doctor's feeling of guilt increases. These families receive more medication and more referrals to hospital outpatient departments than they really need and their problems continue.

Other members of the team have similar difficulties with the same families. The health visitor is defeated by the colicky baby and the untrainable toddler, the nurse treats the verrucae and grazed knees and administers desensitising vaccines, the receptionists are at their wits end trying to find suitable appointments.

In addition to the families who seek frequent medical help, there are those who are only slightly less of a problem and a further group, who do not attend very often, but who nevertheless suffer repeated minor illness and chronic lack of well being. For some families, the standard of health varies within the spectrum at different times. If these groups are added together, we find that a substantial proportion of the population suffers from ill-defined ill health. The average health quotient is low.

The intensity of the problem varies from those women and their families who are overwhelmed by it to those for whom it is an intermittent nuisance, but the healthy woman who only occasionally seeks medical help for herself or her family is becoming a rarity. There is no sign that the management of the situation is improving and it seems likely that the more sophisticated a society becomes, the worse it is. It is clear that we need to look much more closely into its causes if we are to find any solutions.

It is important to remember that these are the majority of the women and children in the practice. They are not a hypochondriacal or neurotic few. They are people with real problems and poor health. They are not shirkers and layabouts trying to get something for nothing. They are people feeling unwell and seeking relief. The fact that they do not often find it, and some have even stopped looking, means that the service we provide is inappropriate to their needs. If that leads us to the conclusion that the training of a doctor is in many ways inappropriate to the needs of general practice, then there is truth in that too.

The Healthy Woman and her Sickly Sister

There are a number of differences between healthy and unhealthy women which taken separately may seem slight but which have an important overall effect. To highlight these differences it is necessary to examine the extremes of the spectrum and to contrast the exceptionally healthy woman with her exceptionally unhealthy counterpart. What have healthy women got that the others lack? They are more confident in themselves and what they are doing. Whether they are full-time wives and mothers, single women with or without children, or working wives, they seem to know that they are doing what is right for them and making a success of it. They have a greater variety of interests and activities both inside the home and outside but there is no common factor in these interests. They are involved with the community. Whatever their special interest, they seem to have more time and energy to spare than do their poorly sisters. When accidents or illness do occur, they are able to cope with them with a minimum of fuss or anxiety. Recovery is rapid, complications few. Their children are rarely absent from school. They have fewer marital problems or at least they cope with them without help. They have little trouble with their neighbours. They have a knack of being pleased with their lot, however poor, and spend little time hankering after what they cannot have or would rather be doing. The self-assurance and self-respect of such a woman is associated with a stable personality, flexible attitudes and a sense of personal security which is not threatened by illness or external events. She has an indestructible inner contentment and joy of living.

What all this adds up to is that these women are happy and it is clear from what happens to the families of happy women over long periods that it is being happy that makes them healthy and not the other way round.

This idea is supported by many studies of how the incidence of disease rises following episodes of stress both in individuals and in communities. The finding of β-haemolytic streptococci in the throats of children could be directly linked with crises in the family.[1] Disease of all sorts is more likely to occur during the two years following a bereavement.[2] There is evidence of an association between levels of unemployment and morbidity and mortality from all causes and at all ages, including infants.[3] It is, therefore, easy to see a link between chronic stress, in the form of unhappiness, and poor health even though it may be difficult to produce statistical data to support the thesis.

Of course, being happy, as well as facilitating good health, also enables a woman to withstand the impact of external stresses on herself and her family. She copes better with financial problems, disappointments and bereavement as well as whatever illness and accidents come her way.

The unhappy woman, already debilitated by her unhappiness and the chronic ill health it causes, will be at even greater risk when crises occur which she cannot resist. She has little self-confidence or self-respect. She dare not trust her own judgement or use her common sense. She is defeated by the most trivial problem or minor illness. In fact she seems defeated by life altogether. She has few interests or activities outside the home and appears bored and anxious within it. Her children, as well as having poor health, behave badly and there are problems with neighbours. She finds it difficult to make friends or get along well with anyone. She has marital problems.

It now becomes clear why a healthy woman has a healthy family. The same personal qualities which enable her to resist disease are passed on to her children from the moment of birth, or even before, and are shared with her husband and other close relations. A crisis in her family passes almost unnoticed. The general daily level of stress is less. The knowledge that his mother is calm, unflappable and flexible enables the child not to worry about her reaction to his missing the bus and being late home, tearing his new clothes or failing to come up to expectations at school. It does not matter if she is cross with him, his position in the family is safe. He can retain his status and self-respect in all circumstances.

The love of his parents is for him as himself and is never conditional on his good behaviour or achievements. With this protective armour, he can cope with any challenge that he is faced with whether to his intellect, emotions or immunological mechanisms. There is evidence that children with happy, healthy mothers are less likely to be involved in road accidents.[4] They have a lower incidence of disease of all sorts.

If any advantage is to be gained from this knowledge, then we must examine why some women are happy and contented with their lot while others are not and what, if anything, the primary health care team can do about it. The causes or roots of happiness, of health, are in many ways more important than the causes of disease.

The Development of a Happy Woman

The most important attributes of the happy woman are her stable personality and sense of security. These allow her to have flexible attitudes to changing circumstances and not to feel threatened or be made anxious by events which upset a woman less well endowed. She quickly adapts to a fall in income, an enforced and unwelcome move to a new area, the failure of a child to pass an exam, or her husband to gain expected promotion. She does not need to have life planned in detail in advance and is not unsettled if plans that are made have to be changed at the last minute.

It is possible that these qualities are to some extent inherited but it is likely that they depend most on the quality of mothering and family life the child experiences from birth onwards and possibly even on prenatal circumstances. They begin to develop in early infancy and can be observed in very young children. They are the result of being brought up by a calm, confident, contented mother, of being consistently loved and valued by both parents, who have a stable, loving relationship with each other, in a settled family, and developing a good long-term relationship with a father or father figure. The mother's state of mind is communicated to the child from birth and possibly even before. The child of the relaxed mother is less likely to have feeding problems or colic, difficulties in sleeping or toilet training. He is thus protected from stresses that he cannot cope with. He faces each stage of development when he is ready for it.

Growing up involves being faced with a series of stressful situations of graded difficulty. If the child deals with a particular challenge successfully, his confidence is strengthened and he is better able to tackle the next and the one after that. In time he will learn to cope with occasional failure. If he is faced with problems which he is not equipped to solve, he will fail, lose confidence and become anxious. A small baby can cope with hunger and thirst provided they are not prolonged. His success in getting them satisfied increases his confidence and contentedness. He cannot cope with an anxious mother, colic or lack of warmth and affection. He will not succeed in dealing with them and will himself become anxious, restless, sleep badly and have more colic.

This process continues throughout childhood and adolescence. A stable family environment, with satisfactory mothering and parental relationships, allows the child to experience difficulties and learn how to cope with them. He is protected from serious problems beyond his capability to handle. He is helped to deal with others. The difficulties he faces gradually become more complex as he grows up but repeated success in dealing with them increases his confidence and expertise. This is maturity.

Other aspects of the happy woman are her self-confidence and self-respect. These stem partly from her mature personality and sense of personal security but they are also related to her position in society. To understand this, it may help to examine briefly the position of women in society.

The Social Position of Women

Despite the rapid changes which are now taking place and the modern fashion for questioning and challenging it, Western society is still firmly established along patriarchal lines. The men are the providers and protectors, the women are the home-makers and care for the children and the men in family units. Sexual roles are well defined and accepted codes of behaviour, social and sexual, are highly developed. This pattern developed thousands of years ago and for good sociological reasons. There were clear advantages in this way of life to the survival and development of the species. Women, or at least some of them, have to bear the children of the community. Until recently, women also had to suckle the children and this process, occupying as it did most of her life, effectively prevented her from doing much else. The family unit and strong sexual taboos with emphasis on the fidelity of the female enabled a man to identify his own children and avoid supporting anyone else's. This was important in evolutionary terms in times when natural selection was a significant force for mankind.

However it is not necessary to look back as far as Greek mythology and stories of the Amazons to discover that women are capable of living and thriving in a wide variety of cultures and of fulfilling greatly differing roles. Margaret Mead, in her studies of Pacific Island cultures, found women as aggressive hunters in one community at the same time as those in another were the organisers and providers and in another were the home-makers and cared for the children. Their attitudes to children ranged from those who would throw the new baby in the river if it were the wrong sex or surplus to requirements, to the closest and most loving relationships in communities where children were the centre of life and of the utmost importance. Attitudes and relationships between the sexes varied equally widely.

In many communities today, children are cared for by the elderly women, either communally or within families, while the young women work and take little part in the domestic chores or the business of making a home. Even within Western societies, there has been a variety in the roles women have played. There has even been a wide range within communities where a woman's lifestyle was determined by her rank and marital status. An upper-class woman might be involved in caring for her family in only a most indirect way. She would employ a wet-nurse, nanny, cook and other domestic staff, her own role being purely supervisory. She might even become an employer, farmer or factory owner in her own right.

The success of the traditional pattern of family life, with the woman's role centred on the home servicing the needs of her family, and the fact that, despite the exceptions, it has been by far the most usual way for human societies to develop, are undeniable, but it clearly owes more to social pressures than to the biological needs of women. There is no characteristic of women which makes this the only way to cultural success. She must bear the children and perhaps suckle them but there is no inborn need in a woman to play a certain role in society, no intrinsic property of womanliness which requires a particular way of life for its fulfilment. Women have physical, intellectual and emotional needs which in every way parallel those of men. How far the differences are innate and how far the result of upbringing is impossible to say. It probably does not matter. They need food and warmth, health and security, to love and be loved, sexual satisfaction, intellectual and physical exercise, status and self-respect. All these needs could be provided for in any one of a variety of situations.

At birth, a female child is totally flexible. She has the potential to fulfil any one of a variety of cultural roles. She could thrive and be happy and healthy in any one of a number of social settings. According to how she is brought up she could be an aggressive protector and provider, a meek and pliant home-maker, a lady of leisure, a leader of men.

A Woman's Health

The manner of her upbringing is all important. She can be nothing without it and yet it is the very thing which limits her capacity to fulfil a diversity of roles. What is most difficult for her is to try, as an adult, to be something other than that for which she has been brought up. By the time she reaches adult life, her flexibility is greatly reduced. From the moment of birth, the process of socialisation shapes her into a member of the class and society into which she is born. She is thereafter capable of functioning satisfactorily only within that class and society.

To survive, human beings must live in groups or communities. In order to do this they have to develop extremely complex patterns of behaviour. No individual can be completely integrated into a community unless she has been through the conditioning process appropriate to that community and her place in it. It is an essential part of growing up, and in adult life the success of the process is a more important factor in the health and happiness of the individual than any biological or inherited characteristic.

The processes of socialisation at present operating in our society are those which have been developed over a number of generations. They vary to some extent between different communities and greatly between classes. They are all geared to stable communities where social changes take place slowly over many generations and where movement between classes and interchange with other very different societies is minimal. A girl growing up in such a community learns from an early age how the society works, what is her place in it and what is expected of her as a member of it.

She learns about family life from personal experience. She observes the behaviour of her parents and the relationship between them. She experiences their attitude towards her, her siblings and each other, and their expectations of her. She learns how to be a wife, mother and member of the community by first of all being a daughter, sister and child within it. The lessons she learns as a child are based on the cultural heritage of her parents and grandparents and only partly on the current facts of life of the society into which she is born. They may bear little relation to the future society in which she will live. If the society is changing rapidly so that by the time she grows up it is very different from the way it was in her parents' and grandparents' time, then the socialisation process to which she was subjected will not have suited her for the life she will lead. She will have difficulties in adjusting to the realities of her situation, whether as wife, mother or employee, and will be subjected to tensions which she may be unable to resolve. The degree of adaptability a woman retains depends upon her personality and this, as has been seen, depends on the quality of her early life.

It is because of the importance of early experience that the uniquely disastrous effect of the Second World War on family life in this country is causing continuing problems. Few families were unaffected by the war. Most children grew up without stable two-parent families and some, the evacuees, without any parents at all for an extended period. Even those families who were eventually reunited experienced tensions which made normal life difficult or impossible. That generation of children had a very distorted model of family life. Many had only a very hazy idea of how to make a marriage work and how to raise children. Added to this was a general atmosphere of unease and insecurity for some years after the war ended. Many men found it difficult to settle down to domesticity on leaving the services. There were rapid technological changes affecting people at home and at work, shortage of housing and pressure on many people to uproot themselves. All these factors combined to make family life unstable, unsatisfying and unhappy. The divorce rate increased and all the same problems were passed on to the next generation — the young parents of today.

Social Strains on Women

Many of the changes in modern society which make life difficult for women are subtle, complex and ill understood. The mobility of the population — about 25 per cent of people move every year in urban communities — has led to the fragmentation of the extended family and the absence for many women of close and supportive ties in the community. Brown and Harris[5] found that women with close friends in the community were less likely to become depressed than those who were socially isolated. There is a much greater strain on a marriage if a woman's husband is her only source of company, comfort and intellectual stimulation. She is likely to have greater difficulty in bringing up her children if she has no peer group of other mothers with whom to compare notes, share problems and measure herself and her family by. The mechanisation of much housework, full-time education and small, closely spaced families, have meant that women have a great deal of time which is not required to service the needs of the family. Those who find satisfying jobs outside the home certainly seem happier,[6] but for a woman to take a full-time job places her and her family under enormous strain, and part-time work is scarce, of poor quality and status, and poorly paid. Even for those with training or special skills, it is difficult to obtain work consistent with their aptitudes and abilities and most women marry and start a family without undergoing any

A Woman's Health

training, or developing any special skills. A further problem is that a woman working outside the home is more likely to neglect relationships within the community and may become even more socially isolated than others who do not have jobs but work at developing and continuing local friendships and activities.

Changes in recent years have meant that girls have left school with a higher expectation of life than previous generations. They expect more action, more excitement and a more interesting and satisfying life than did their mothers or grandmothers. There is less emphasis on survival and more on fulfilment. The problem is that education has not succeeded in equipping most women with the ability to achieve these ambitions and society makes it difficult for them to do so.

Whether more by nature or nurture, healthy women are emotionally more liberated, able to love and be loved more freely than men and with less inhibition. They are capable of greater intensity in their relationships as lovers and as mothers. They are physically more resilient, less likely to suffer disability or premature death and have greater reserves of strength and resourcefulness which they can summon up in an emergency. Many of them have had an extended training in home-building and child care during their own early life. They are therefore ideally equipped to provide the stable home base, which children and men need. This is what the vast majority want to do but in doing it they also want the excitement, stimulation and satisfaction which men are supposed to find in their lives outside the home. By devaluing the work of the wife and mother, society has made it difficult for most women to see it as the worthwhile job it should be. Even men who have boring and seemingly futile jobs at least have the satisfaction of bringing home a wage packet. This is very important in a materialistic society. The woman with no wage packet, no job satisfaction, no status and little self-respect rapidly becomes demoralised. She then fails to do the work as well as she might and sinks still further.

Maintaining Self-respect

A great deal depends on every woman developing and maintaining an idea of her own value and her role in society outside her marriage and family. For a woman to deny her own individuality, her own need for friends, interests and fulfilment, and to make herself first and only a wife and mother places intolerable strains on her marriage and family. It is unusual for any marital relationship to be so intense and satisfying as to fulfil the entire emotional and intellectual needs of both partners. Even when it does, the death of one or other is more totally shattering than it need be had the relationship been more normal. Most married women eventually become widows. Many live as widows for twenty or thirty years. Their happiness during this period depends entirely on their ability to integrate into the community and they are unlikely to be able to achieve such integration if they were isolated from society during the years of their marriage.

More commonly, happy and successful marriages are those in which both partners have equally important interests both within and outside the home, where there is mutual recognition of the equal value of each and of the work each does. The wife may run the home and care for the children, find company in the local young wives group and intellectual stimulation at an evening class while her husband finds all these in an exciting and well-paid job. Both have to realise that what she does is as important as what he does. Society as a whole must also recognise the importance of child care and home-making as jobs whether they are done by men or women. We need a re-examination of all our values, a recognition of the worth of each individual as a member of society regardless of what he does. The fact that 'Do you work?' — 'No, I am only a housewife' is a daily and unremarked interchange is an indictment of our society.

For some women, life certainly does come up to their expectations. For others, there are good times and bad. For many, life consists of long periods of disappointment, disillusion and depression. Which of these groups a woman finds herself in seems to depend more on her own background, personality and natural drive than on external forces, but there are many who would succeed in living happy, fulfilled lives if not too many difficulties lie in their way or if a helping hand is offered from time to time. The help she needs can come from a variety of sources and in many different guises. Its most appropriate form will depend on the nature of the woman's problem and also on her personality and situation. The problem itself may be something she can handle herself or which will be resolved provided she has support and comfort. The more closely integrated she is with the community, the more likely she is to have friends who will help her through a crisis or foresee problems and help to lessen their impact. Many women find this kind of close integration difficult and in most modern communities a large proportion of the families have only recently arrived and have few or no close contacts. However mobile the population, in every community there is a nucleus of organisations and people who can provide continuity of community life and try to ensure that newcomers are drawn into it as soon, and as completely, as possible. This nucleus is made up of a number of different elements and is unique to each community. The churches, schools, pubs and local shops all play a part as also, to a greater or lesser extent, do outposts of the social services department and voluntary organisations. The success of the community depends upon the loose and unorganised way in which these various strands function, working separately but pulling together.

The primary health care team can form an important element in this network. Its particular contribution is to link the other strands and to work with them and through them, as well as on its own, to promote the happiness and the health of the community, to prevent disease as far as can be done and to help the community to manage such disease as does occur, minimising misery and speeding recovery when this is possible, easing death when it is not. Its especial aim is to raise the health quotient of the individual members of the community.

There are those who say that this is not the job of the primary health care team; that social work should be done by the social services department, that doctors and their attached staff should stick to medicine: that is, to diagnosing and treating disease. This is no longer a tenable point of view. It is not possible to separate healthy people and sick people into compartments, to treat disease without also trying to prevent it, or to treat disease without considering those factors which delay recovery.

About half of the work at present done by general practitioners is in comforting people with minor, self-limiting sickness and reassuring those with trivial symptoms and no treatable disease. The present service is overstretched and unable to cope with its workload. Society cannot afford, and probably ought not to spend, a higher proportion of its resources on health care. If the average health quotient of the population could be raised, there would be less illness of all kinds. If, at the same time, it were possible to increase the ability of the community and its individual members to manage minor illness and symptoms without professional help and to share in the treatment of other disease to a greater extent, then the present allocation of resources might be adequate.

Doctors cannot effect these changes but primary health care teams might be able to. There are no other agencies with the necessary central and universal position in the community which could even attempt it. It has to be accepted that the promotion of health and prevention and treatment of disease are the responsibility of the primary health care team, and the promotion of happiness and health in women should be their starting-point.

Notes

1. R.J. Meyer and R.J. Haggerty, 'Steptococcal Infections in Families', *Pediatrics*, vol. 29 (1962), p. 539.

2. C.M. Parkes, 'Broken Heart: A Statistical Study of Increased Mortality among Widowers', *British Medical Journal*, vol. 1 (1969), p. 740; W.D. Rees and S.G. Lutkins, 'Mortality and Bereavement', *British Medical Journal*, vol. 4 (1967), p. 13; D. Maddison and A.J. Viola, 'The Health of Widows in the year following Bereavement', *Psychosomatic Research*, vol. 12 (1968), p. 297.

3. A.R. Bunn and N.T. Drane, *New Doctor*, vol. 5 (1977), p. 53; M.H. Brenner, *Estimating the Social Costs of National Economic Policy* (US Government Printing Office, 1976).

4. G.W. Brown and S. Davidson, 'Social Class. Psychiatric Disorder of Mother, and Accidents to Children', *Lancet*, vol. 1 (1978), p. 378.

5. G.W. Brown and T. Harris, *Social Origins of Depression* (Tavistock Publications, London, 1978).

6. Ibid.

2 THE ROLE OF THE PRIMARY HEALTH CARE TEAM

There is nothing the members of the primary health care team can do about a woman's upbringing, once she is an adult, but there are things which can be done to counteract some of its bad effects and they may be able to influence the upbringing and future health of children. Therefore their work in this area can be roughly divided into two parts: ameliorating the present problems of women and preventing similar problems arising in the next generation. These two parts are closely linked and overlap because, to a great extent, the problems of one generation are the direct result of those of the one before, so that, if life can be improved for present-day mothers, then the future prospects for their children are immediately better.

While most women do not have all the qualities of the ideal, happy woman described in Chapter 1, most do have some of them and can be encouraged to develop them. Self-confidence and competence are important among these. A woman has the main responsibility for the way the members of her family live. She regulates what everyone eats, whether the house is clean and tidy, how the children behave, when they go to bed, get up, go to school. She is also in charge of sickness. She makes the first diagnosis, chooses and carries out treatment and decides whether and when to seek outside help and from whom. If she sees a doctor, she has to present the problem to him, understand what he says and understand and carry out his advice. All this amounts to a heavy responsibility, requiring skill and knowledge to discharge. The burden of it causes anxiety in many women. There are a number of ways in which this anxiety can be lessened and self-confidence increased. Modern society has built up an inflated view of the value of the professional whether he be a teacher, doctor, child psychologist or anything else. This has had the effect of undermining the confidence of many women in their own judgement and ability to cope. They are often treated as idiots by experts and their staff whether at the local garage, school or doctor's surgery and in fact they sometimes do lack the knowledge which would make everyday life easier for them.

How the Health Team Can Help

The first task of the members of the primary health care team is to make sure that nothing in their attitude to the patient could in any way further undermine her self-confidence. She should be treated with respect however silly she may seem. They should show respect for her, for her way of life and for the decisions she makes. If anyone offers advice, it should always be worded in such a way that it does not suggest that what she is doing is wrong. All advice should be in the form of 'you may like to try' rather than 'you must do'. She should be left with the clear idea that it is up to her to decide whether to accept it or not. Only she can tell whether it is the advice she needs and can use with advantage. Her opinion is ultimately the only one that matters.

Next, the primary health care team can provide information. The mother may not be able to treat a child with a cold simply because she does not know how. Information should be freely available on many subjects, from how to make an appointment at the surgery, to toilet training, and in several different forms: leaflets, posters, booklets, talks, word of mouth. A booklet can be very useful, with charts or lists of various common symptoms and how they may be treated and suggestions as to when to ask for professional advice. It is a great help if members of the team are easily available on the telephone to discuss problems of minor illness. The woman can be encouraged in her management of the case, suggestions made to help her and unnecessary home visits avoided. Practices where a doctor is available in this way at weekends, find themselves doing far fewer home visits than those using a telephone answering service.

Groups of mothers, such as those whose children attend a nursery school, or the members of a mother and toddler group, can be encouraged to invite a member of the team to come and join a discussion about health topics. Anxiety about infectious diseases, toilet training and feeding and sleeping problems can be lessened by such meetings.

A great deal is learnt by example. If a mother takes a child with a cold to the doctor and he gives her a prescription, she will have learnt that when a child gets a cold he should be taken to the doctor and receive medication. It makes no difference what the doctor says or what the medication is. It may take longer for him to explain to her how she can treat the child herself but it will enable her to manage on her own next time. The best thing of all is for the doctor to ask the mother what she is already doing and say something like 'I cannot improve on that, you are already doing all that can be done.' A health visitor in a well-baby clinic can teach the mother a lot by the way she handles and talks to a child. Receptionists frequently teach in this way:

The Role of the Primary Health Care Team 27

'No, there are no appointments today unless it is an emergency.'
'He has tummyache and vomiting.'
'Wait and I will fit you in in a minute.'

A mother may be better able to cope with family life if she has regular contact with other women with families so that she can compare her experience with theirs. She may copy good ideas and reject aspects of their way of life which she dislikes. She will be able to form an idea of what is normal. She will be able to congratulate herself on some things and resolve to change others. The knowledge that other people have similar difficulties is itself helpful. The health visitor should know about women's clubs, mother and toddler groups or even individual neighbours to whom she can introduce a particular woman. She should also be able to help fill any gaps in her knowledge of child-rearing and the management of minor illness. She may be able to provide leaflets on some subjects. In all her dealings with the woman she should demonstrate her respect for her as a person and for her capabilities as a wife and mother.

The Patient's Responsibility

A major fault of medical practice in recent years has been the way in which it has tried to take over responsibility for illness and its management from the patient. The authoritarian, paternalistic doctor makes decisions for the patient 'in his best interest' and issues instructions for him to carry out, assuming, without question, that the patient can, and will, do as he is told and benefit thereby. A great deal of illness is treated in hospital where the patient behind the illness is largely ignored. Outpatient appointments are arranged at intervals to be decided by the specialist with no reference to the patient's view of his needs. Even dying now usually takes place in hospital and is something which the staff do for the patient. Many people seem to die as people as soon as they are even admitted for terminal care. Some people do not mind being treated like this, but even for those the system does not work efficiently. Even within the confines of the traditional medical practice, the doctor needs the active and informed co-operation of the patient at all stages. They must work together as partners if they are to achieve the best results. It is of no use treating the illness without treating the patient.

Doctors are trained to diagnose and treat disease. They make a diagnosis by listening to the story the patient presents, asking questions and carrying out an examination if necessary. They treat an illness perhaps by giving the patient a prescription and some instructions.

Many conscientious doctors see this as the limit of their responsibility. They fail to realise that their diagnosis is based on the patient's understanding of what the doctor needs to know and that the most important part of the history is often not revealed. The resulting diagnosis is likely to be inaccurate or irrelevant. They also overlook the fact that it is not the doctor who treats the illness but the woman herself who does so with the benefit of the doctor's advice. If, as often happens, she fails to understand or remember the advice or what to expect from the medication, the treatment is not in fact carried out as the doctor believes it will be.

Listening to the Patient

The only way a doctor can make sure that he obtains the history relevant to the woman's real problem is for him to be constantly on the lookout for signs that she has something else to say and to beware of jumping to the first diagnosis that presents itself. Whenever a patient enters the consulting room, the doctor has a slight feeling of anxiety that he is not going to know what is wrong with her or her child and is going to be unable to satisfy her demands. If her opening remarks enable him to make a diagnosis, it is tempting for him to grasp the opportunity, not realising that even if it is a correct diagnosis, it may not be the most important one or the problem which most urgently needs attention. The child may indeed have asthma but if the doctor fails to discover the mother's anxiety, which is related to quite another matter, but which is an important factor in the child's asthma, his treatment will be ineffective.

The old adage that, if you listen to the patient, she will give you the diagnosis, is absolutely true but you have to listen to everything the patient says and to heed a lot of non-verbal signals too. The doctor should always assume that things are not what they seem.

Informing the Patient

Many women attend the doctor to ask his opinion. They often do not want him to treat them, do not want medicines and are quite prepared for the illness to take its course or to put up with symptoms which have no sinister significance. Doctors are far too ready to prescribe medicines and even physiotherapy for patients who do not really need them. Few ever ask a woman whether she would like treatment for the condition. Most illnesses and all of the undiagnosable malaises can be satisfactorily managed in a number of different ways. There is no one 'right way'. When there is no clear clinical indication for a particular form of management, it is only reasonable to put the alternatives before the patient and let her choose. One of these alternatives should always be to use no drugs. If a woman is to administer treatment, she must want to do so and she must understand and accept the need for it. Whatever the decision, for the management of the illness to succeed, the woman should be openly acknowledged as an essential partner and of at least equal importance to the doctor. She needs the following information:

About the Illness

What is the likely course of the illness in terms of length and of symptoms? How serious is it?
Are there any symptoms which should be reported to the doctor?
Under what circumstances should she return to the doctor or ask him to call?
Should the patient stay in bed – all day, part of the day? lie flat? avoid any particular activity? stay indoors? avoid contact with other people? lead a normal life?
Should the patient have a special diet?
If she is referred to a hospital specialist, she should be encouraged to return to the general practitioner to discuss his findings and explain his advice.
If investigations are to be carried out, she should be told when to expect the results and what to do about them.

About the Medication

How should the drug be given? i.e. by what route – how often – when in relation to meals – for how long – is it a short course or should it be continued indefinitely?
What effect is it likely to have on the illness? – immediate cure, delayed cure, no visible effect?
Should the drug be continued after the cessation of the symptoms?
If the drug is to be given 'as required' exactly what is the indication for a dose? How often may it be repeated? What is the maximum total dose in 24 hours?
What side effects – are to be expected – are likely – are possible, but nothing to worry about – should be reported to the doctor – should make her stop the drug?

If a child of five develops whooping cough, the doctor will save himself a lot of trouble and the mother much anxiety if he tells her that it is not serious at this age; is likely to last a total of about six weeks, but that the cough alone may continue or recur for a long time after that and that the child need not stay in bed but should be kept away from other children for three weeks after the onset of the whoop. The child should be brought to see him again after an arranged interval. In the meantime the mother should let him know if the child becomes ill or has difficulty in breathing between the paroxysms. If he prescribes an antibiotic, he should explain that it will probably not affect the course of the illness but may protect the child against other infection during it. The course should be completed but not repeated and should be stopped if a rash appears. He should not criticise her for not having had the child immunised. He should suggest she telephones him if she is at all anxious.

An immediate problem with this sort of information is that it is difficult to retain. There are several ways to help a woman to remember what has been said. The doctor can ask her to repeat back the most important items; he can write down a short version of some of it while he is saying it and she then takes the piece of paper with her as an aide-de-memoire; he can provide her with a leaflet about the condition or treatment or a list or chart on which he only has to mark certain relevant items; a nurse can see the woman on her way out and explain and reinforce what the doctor has said and make sure the patient understands and accepts it. She may be able to answer further questions the woman has. The doctor should make clear in the patient's notes what advice he has given so that the receptionist may repeat it to her if she returns later to check on any point.

Establishing Medical Records

The primary health care team is in a particularly advantageous position to identify women who are at especial risk and to protect them from its consequences. If this is to be done efficiently the practice needs good medical records, each of which contains basic data about the patient, a commitment to the work by all members, a high level of 'useful gossip' and an agreed pattern of responsibility.

The basic data about each patient should be entered on a special sheet not used for anything else. It can be obtained by asking the woman to complete a short questionnaire for each member of her family when she first registers. For people already registered with the practice, the details can be obtained at their next visit to the surgery. Information required:

Name, address, date of birth.
Previous address and name of doctor.

Names of other members of the household.
Family history: ages of parents, siblings, children and date, age and cause of death where appropriate.
Personal history: occupation, smoking habits, height and weight.
Medical history: Illnesses, accidents, operations. Any current medication?
Menstrual and obstetric history: Do you have regular periods? If not, when did they stop?
Do you have bleeding between periods?
Are you taking an oral contraceptive?
Have you had any pregnancies? (If so, please give details, including dates of confinement/miscarriage and weights of babies.)
Have you had any of the following tests and if so was the result satisfactory?
    Blood pressure.
    Urine test.
    Chest X-ray.
    Cervical smear.

The questionnaire can be adapted to include anything that the members of the primary health care team think important. Immediately it reveals a great deal of information which may be useful from the disease-prevention point of view. Any obese, heavy smoker who has not had her blood pressure taken and whose father died at forty from a coronary would be identified and could be offered an appointment to have her serum lipids and blood pressure taken even if she declines advice on her weight and smoking. If a woman reports intermenstrual or post-menopausal bleeding, she could be invited to visit the doctor about it.

In addition to these purely medical facts, those families with a lot of illness, recent bereavements, many young children, disabled members or only one parent, will be identified, as will women living alone or in lodgings. The high level of useful gossip will reveal much significant information which the team can put to good use. Which firms are laying off staff? Whose husband has left home? Who has been killed/injured in an accident, taken an overdose or been up in court for not paying the rates? Has the barmaid, who snapped at the receptionist in the pub, defaulted on her phenothiazine injection? If she has, and can be chased up by the community psychiatric nurse, a serious and prolonged illness perhaps involving danger to life, admission to hospital under a section of the Mental Health Act and even electro-convulsive therapy, may be avoided. Who is beating their children, drinking heavily or coming to the surgery more often or for trivial reasons? The receptionist is often the key figure in all this. Only she knows that Mrs Green has telephoned the health visitor, doctor, social worker and nurse separately during a few days, each for an apparently minor problem, and is obviously under stress. She is in a unique position to observe how people behave in the waiting room, where family relationships are often strained and the mother's patience exhausted. She can pass on to the doctor the intense panic and anguish behind a request for a visit, emotions which are often suppressed when he arrives at the house.

It is obviously necessary to guard against irrelevant scandal-mongering. The balance is a nice one and often difficult to keep. It should be an aspect of their work which the members of the team discuss together and help each other with.

Who Needs Help?

Having identified a woman who is particularly at risk, either because of her inadequate personality, awful circumstances or a recent disaster, it has to be decided whether she needs help and who, if anyone, should offer it. The woman may decide for herself by contacting a member of the team or she may be known to be an active member of a church group and unlikely to need further support. Someone in the team has to be responsible for co-ordinating the information and action or it may be done jointly at a regular meeting.

It will always be the particular responsibility of the health visitor to watch for signs of post-natal depression in a mother with a child under a year old but it may in fact be the receptionist or surgery nurse who first suspects it and sometimes a neighbour or the local vicar who will express their concern. The problem may be resolved by a visit from the health visitor and perhaps grandmother coming to stay for a few days, or it may need doctor, community psychiatric nurse and social worker as well before all aspects of the illness and its effects on the rest of the family are examined and the total misery reduced to a minimum.

Some families are happiest and thrive best if the mother goes out to work and employs a nanny or childminder to care for her children for part of the time. The financial advantage may not be significant but if this arrangement results in a happier, more fulfilled woman then the whole family will benefit. It helps no one for such a woman to persist in her attempts to be a full-time wife and mother out of a sense of duty if to do so makes her unhappy, irritable, frustrated and depressed. She will be a better mother and have more successful family relationships if she is encouraged to live her own life to the full. Everyone should avoid criticism of a woman in this situation and every help and support should be offered her for the benefit of her happiness and health.

If offered encouragement, help, support and opportunities at the right time to carry them through crises and difficult periods in their lives, many women, who would otherwise have drifted, with their children, into chronic ill health, may be enabled to live lives approaching those of the ideal women abounding with health, vigour, energy, enthusiasm and happiness.

Working in Schools

If the primary health care team is fully integrated into the life of the community and responsible for the whole of health care, its members will have opportunities to visit and work in schools. This field is largely unexplored but it may prove possible to influence attitudes and values among both teachers and children so that self-respect, the value of the individual and the status of women become as important as academic standards. There is evidence that some teachers already lean in this direction[1] but are constantly under pressure from parents to demonstrate their enthusiasm for intellectual achievement to the exclusion of all else. The irony is that, if a child is happy and confident, her intellectual capacity is more likely to be used to the full. As with health, the ability to learn depends on self-respect and a high sense of one's own value. These can be encouraged by teachers even in children who lack a secure, loving home background. At present far more boys than girls stay on at school and seek academic qualifications and training after they leave school. They have a greater motivation to do so because the need is obvious: they must earn a living. They also have greater self-respect. To girls the need is not so obvious. For many of them, marriage is enough of a goal unless the desirability of other objectives is made very clear to them. Girls with a high self-regard and sense of status are more likely to stay on after the school-leaving age and seek qualifications, training or higher education, than those who put a low value on themselves. They will be less likely to marry young and more likely to retain their own interests and individuality if and when they do marry. The quality of life for them will be higher whether they marry or have children or not. This is an important factor in the health of the next generation.

There are many opportunities for co-operation with schools over individual children with problems, which are at present being neglected. Teachers and members of the primary health care team are in a position to forecast at an early age which children are likely to have serious difficulties in adolescence or adult life and yet at present nothing is done about such children unless or until they become a nuisance either within school or in the community at large. Then it is usually only those who are delinquent or who fail to attend school who are offered help. This help comes much too late to be of any use, often several years after the first signs of disturbance or unhappiness appear and it is only offered to those whose misery leads them into antisocial or non-conformist behaviour. This means that most unhappy girls receive no help. Their reaction to their problems is more often depression than anger and this does not get them into trouble. They fail to fulfil their potential at school and are held in low regard by their parents, their teachers and, most importantly, by themselves. They are the next generation of unhappy, unhealthy mothers of unhappy, unhealthy families.

The sort of co-operation needed to effect any change in the outlook for children with difficulties would have to start when the children start school and would have to be enthusiastically supported by both the teachers and the members of the primary health care team. This may be difficult to achieve. At a recent meeting to discuss plans in this field a primary school headmaster said: 'We do not need help from the child guidance clinic with difficult children in our school. We can handle them.' He and many of his colleagues clearly felt it was an admission of failure on their part to ask for help for a child. Most people see the only reason for trying to help a child as being an inability to contain him in school or the community. If the criteria of future health and learning ability were used instead, then it might be possible to offer help to children at an early age when it could have some effect.

As well as these broad considerations, there are areas in the lives of women which are particularly likely to give rise to stress and which may afford the primary health care team opportunities to extend its work in the prevention of ill health in the community. Some of these will be examined in the chapters which follow.

Notes

1. P.E. Daunt, *Comprehensive Values* (Heinemann, London, 1975).

3 MENSTRUATION

Menstruation gives rise to a great deal of anxiety among women. It is universal and yet it is surrounded by ignorance and mystery. Many professional health workers are ill informed on the subject. It is a process which is subject to wide fluctuations of normal as well as producing symptoms associated with disease and so it is important first to consider what is normal.

The Normal Menstrual Cycle

As with all other bodily functions, normality means different things to different people. The range is wide and it is difficult for any individual woman to know what it is. There is no well-recognised standard against which she can measure her own pattern. The symptoms that a woman brings to a doctor will depend on her own previous experience, on information she may have picked up from relatives, friends or magazines, and on other problems she may have at the time. All that can be said about the normal menstrual cycle is that it consists of a period of bleeding of variable length and amount, followed by a longer time when there is no bleeding.

The length of the cycle is the time from the first day of one period to the first day of the next. When asked the length of the cycle most women will answer with the time clear between periods. This leads to confusion. It is important for a doctor to understand what he is being told. The length of the normal cycle is variable and it may be different at different times. It is normal for some women to start a period regularly every 28 days. It is equally normal for others to have a regular 50-day cycle. For some women the normal cycle is never regular so that the length may be 25 days on some occasions and 60 on others.

For many women the pattern changes from time to time. There may be a temporary change as happens under stress, or long-term changes in pattern may occur. These are not symptoms of gynaecological disease, although they may be evidence of emotional problems.

It is extremely difficult to measure or describe the amount and length of bleeding. Most doctors are guided by the number of tampons or sanitary towels used each month: 10-15 is common, 30 is a lot. This is not very reliable as some women change more frequently than others.

An apparently normal uterus may bleed heavily as a result of hormonal influences. Whether such bleeding is unacceptably excessive depends on the woman's attitude and lifestyle as much as on the actual volume of blood lost. Working-class women will put up with much heavier bleeding than will middle-class women. Some young intellectual career women so resent menstruating at all that a relatively small loss will seem excessive to them.

The length of the period also varies from two to three days to a week or more. Again this is a question of degree and acceptability rather than normality. There is no absolute standard of normality. Most doctors will consider bleeding to be excessive if it results in anaemia despite a normal diet, or if clots form, or if it interferes with a woman's normal activities. Even these criteria are not strictly indicative of abnormality but more of unacceptability. Even severe menorrhagia is not often associated with organic disease of the uterus.

Most women accept as normal a certain amount of cramp-like lower abdominal pain or backache during the first day or two of menstruation. It should respond to simple analgesics like aspirin or paracetamol and should not interfere with normal activities.

It is common to experience swings of mood corresponding to the menstrual cycle. The usual pattern is for a woman to feel at her lowest during the week before a period starts. She may be more irritable, emotionally labile, clumsy and tired. She may have a slightly bloated feeling and even put on several pounds in weight due to fluid retention.

The only criterion of normality common to all women is that there should be no bleeding between the periods. Normal menstruation may be scanty or profuse, regular or irregular, painless or painful, but each episode should be finite.

The definition of normal may seem vague but there is an even vaguer group of symptoms associated with menstruation which cannot be considered normal and yet are not associated with diagnosable disease. They especially affect the unhappy, unhealthy group of women with a low health quotient identified in Chapter 1. They are not hysterical or neurotic. They are real and distressing but they are still in certain respects physiological. They reflect the body's response to stress and not to disease.

Dysmenorrhoea

Painful periods are not a sign of sinister disease but may be anything from a minor irritation to an incapacitating nuisance. Dysmenorrhoea is most common in young girls within the first three or four years after the onset of menstruation. It may be a constant dull ache in the lower abdomen or back, starting the day before bleeding starts (congestive dysmenorrhoea), or sharp, intermittent pains or colic on the first day (spasmodic dysmenorrhoea). It may be accompanied by nausea, vomiting, headache, dizziness or backache. It can be very severe and it is not surprising that many young women seek help from their doctors for it. What is less obvious is the reason why doctors find it so difficult to be helpful. No one really understands the mechanism of dysmenorrhoea. A doctor may recognise that it has emotional undertones and know that it is unlikely to be a symptom of organic disease. It is not therefore medically interesting. He knows there is very little he can do to relieve it. He feels inadequate when confronted with it. His main idea is to get the patient with dysmenorrhoea out of the consulting room as quickly as possible with a minimum of ill feeling. The patient is likely to be aware of the doctor's resentment and feel that the complaint is not being taken seriously. Often both parents will accompany a quite mature young woman to the doctor to reinforce her description of the symptoms and he will feel all the more irritated. Much of this can be avoided if the doctor can manage to be truly sympathetic and completely honest. He may even save himself time in reducing future visits. He needs to accept completely the patient's description of the symptoms and to show enough interest to elucidate further details that she may have failed to give. He should ask and note her age, the date of onset of her periods, length of the cycle during the past six months and the length of each period. He should elicit details of the pain. Does it occur every month? Where is it? Is it constant or colicky? How long does it last? When did it start? What relieves it? What makes it worse? What has she tried for it? Is she, or should she be, using contraception? Is there any vaginal discharge between the periods? What is the bowel function like (a) usually and (b) just before the period? Are there any symptoms other than pain, e.g. nausea, vomiting, headache? Questions about emotional stress must be asked but it is important to realise that the girl may interpret them as a suggestion that the pain is imaginary. If she does, she will be angry and resentful and impossible to help. Something like, 'I have noticed that girls often find period pains worse when they are worried or upset, have you noticed that?' may make it easier.

A woman recently brought her daughter aged fifteen to the surgery complaining of crippling dysmenorrhoea. We had the usual preliminary talk and then I said: 'I wonder how you get on with your father? I have noticed that a girl's periods have often started being painful if her relationship with her father deteriorates.' There was a vaguely negative response from them both and they left agreeing to try some simple remedies and come again in three months. A few days later the mother returned alone. She said that things were very bad at home. She and her husband were not getting on well and he nagged the girl constantly ('never has a kind word to say to her'). It turned out that the girl's painful periods were a symptom of the family's problems and were relieved when she realised this. There seems no doubt there is a causal relationship between emotional stress and dysmenorrhoea. The fact that no one really understands what it is is no excuse for ignoring or denying it. There is often some anxiety with sexual connotations such as difficulty in establishing sexual identity, poor relationship with father, or fear of pregnancy. However, this is by no means always the case. Menstruation is affected by any sort of stress and in many ways. In a healthy woman, periods may become heavier or lighter, more frequent or less, shorter or more prolonged, painful or totally absent as a result of emotional strain.

Sometimes it is enough for the doctor to have discussed all aspects of the problem and shown understanding and sympathy. A vaginal examination is indicated only if the symptoms add up to more than simple dysmenorrhoea or if the girl herself is anxious that there is something physically wrong with her. It may be that simple measures will suffice. If analgesia is necessary, it is important that it is taken as soon as possible after the onset of pain, or even an hour or two before, if it can be forecast. It must then be repeated every four hours during the time that pain can be expected. Aspirin (two, four-hourly) is probably the most effective and safest of the simple analgesics available and least likely to produce side-effects. However, if it is not tolerated, then paracetamol is a possible alternative. Dextropropoxyphene hydrochloride may also be used but care should be taken not to give it for too long as it appears that it is sometimes addictive and it causes drowsiness in a number of people. If nausea or vomiting are a problem, prochlorperazine ('Stemetil') may be helpful. Some women find that they tend to be constipated during the few days before a period and dysmenorrhoea is sometimes relieved by using a laxative at this time. It is widely known both amongst doctors and patients that the contraceptive pill often relieves dysmenorrhoea. Some girls will approach the doctor hoping to be put on the pill, concealing the request behind a complaint of painful periods. If this appears to be a possibility, the doctor should mention the contraceptive pill as one of the ways of helping dysmenorrhoea even if only to explain why he does not feel it is appropriate on this occasion. It certainly does not seem to be a good idea to put a young girl on the pill purely for the treatment of dysmenorrhoea within the first few years of the menarche, or at least until the menstrual cycle is well established.

At the end of the consultation, the doctor and patient should agree a plan for dealing with the problem for the next three to four months. This may include keeping a menstrual chart, which the doctor should provide, and taking analgesics in a prearranged way. The girl should be asked to return at the end of this time and discuss the situation. The effect of this is to make her realise that the problem is being taken seriously, that the doctor is interested and is doing something. She is unlikely to return sooner than the arranged date.

Throughout this section, it has been assumed that the doctor is the member of the primary health care team to whom this problem is brought. In fact it may well be that a practice nurse would be a better person to deal with it. The management could be exactly the same.

Listening to the Patient

When a woman enters the surgery the doctor can have no idea exactly why she has come. When she starts describing her periods he may be very little nearer finding out. If she is at all diffident or inarticulate, and he impatient, he may never discover. He cannot possibly help her unless he does, so this is an area well worth studying. From a purely technical point of view, the diagnosis and further investigation depend on an accurate history. A woman complains of irregular bleeding which on careful elucidation turns out to be a normal, if erratic, menstrual cycle with no sinister symptoms. She has come because it represents a change from her previous pattern. Perhaps she has been having an affair with a man at work and has been worried about possible pregnancy, her husband finding out, and the break-up of the marriage. There are problems in the marriage because of her husband's inept lovemaking. The impatient doctor fails to elicit anything more than the initial complaint of irregular bleeding. Anxious, quite rightly, not to miss a serious diagnosis of organic disease, he refers her to a gynaecologist for a D & C. A few months later she returns with further symptoms of stress.

A woman may know that irregular bleeding is an important symptom without knowing exactly what it is. She comes to the doctor with what is in fact only a change from one normal menstrual pattern to another. In reassuring her that the symptom is not sinister he should explain how menstrual patterns vary under stress, so that she has an opportunity to ask for help in this area if she needs it. He should also explain what true 'irregular bleeding' is and confirm that she is correct in thinking it should be investigated. If he fails to do this, his reassurance is useless

Amenorrhoea

The onset of menstruation is the last of the signs of puberty to appear. It is preceded by breast development, the appearance of pubic and axillary hair and a rapid growth spurt. Parents often seek advice about girls whose periods have failed to appear. If the whole of puberty is delayed the doctor has to decide whether this particular girl is normal but developing slowly or whether there is an endocrine abnormality. This may be very difficult. Sometimes there may be associated physical signs such as the webbed neck of Turner's Syndrome or a clue may be found in the family history. The mother or her sisters may have had a physiologically late menarche. Most girls have started to menstruate by the age of fifteen so that if there are no signs of puberty by then it would seem reasonable to start investigations. If all other signs of puberty are present except menstruation, it is essential to exclude cryptomenorrhoea due to an imperforate hymen or vaginal septum. Once this is done it is reasonable to wait for several years or even until the woman desires pregnancy before investigating further.

Pregnancy is the commonest cause of secondary amenorrhoea whatever the history volunteered by the patient. Full penetration is not necessary for impregnation and a girl who believes she has taken no risks and still has an intact hymen may nevertheless conceive if contact has been close at the moment of ejaculation. A pregnancy test and vaginal examination should be done not earlier than six weeks after the first day of the last menstrual period and repeated a month later if they are negative.

In women under twenty-five, anorexia nervosa is a common cause of amenorrhoea. Menstruation may stop within a week or two of starting to diet and before weight loss is obvious. Mild forms of anorexia nervosa are very common. The amenorrhoea may persist for many months after the girl has apparently reverted to a normal diet and without her having lost a lot of weight or become abnormally thin. It is important to continue to observe these women and to make sure they have no serious psychiatric symptoms or emotional difficulties with which they need help. Very often the situation resolves itself. More florid cases of anorexia nervosa need the help of a psychiatrist.

The menstrual cycle is often erratic during the first two to three years after the menarche and it is common for young women to menstruate at intervals of several months before a regular cycle is established. Even after a regular cycle has been established, many women develop temporary amenorrhoea in response to stress or sometimes for no obvious reason. Help with emotional problems may be indicated and it is clearly important to exclude physical diseases such as hypothyroidism, hypopituarism or general debilitating diseases such as diabetes mellitus or tuberculosis – not uncommon in immigrants.

Menstruation usually restarts within six to eight weeks of a confinement if a woman does not breast feed. If she does, then the cycle may not be re-established until she stops lactating.

Some women taking oral contraceptives do not have withdrawal bleeding during the pill-free weeks. This does not matter as long as pregnancy and other important causes of amenorrhoea have been excluded and the woman herself does not mind. Some women welcome this situation but many feel it is in some way unhealthy or that the menstrual fluid is still being produced and is collecting somewhere inside. If she is worried about it, it is worth trying a different pill or stopping oral contraceptives. Post-pill amenorrhoea is a common phenomenon. Normal menstruation usually takes six to eight weeks to be re-established after stopping an oral contraceptive, but it is often longer and sometimes the amenorrhoea is prolonged for several years. It is only a serious problem if the woman wants to conceive, when endocrinological help may be necessary.

Mood Change During the Menstrual Cycle

If a woman is under stress or suffers from chronic low-grade misery, then the normal fluctuations of mood during the menstrual cycle may produce marked depression, anxiety or irritability during the premenstrual week. It seems unlikely that so-called pre-menstrual tension will produce these symptoms in a woman who is otherwise well and happy but it does seem to have the effect of making her less able to cope with stress, more vulnerable and therefore exaggerates symptoms which she already has but can cover up at other times. It is fashionable to give progestogen tablets, progesterone pessaries or pyridoxine tablets during the second half of each cycle, and one of these may be helpful, but it is important that the significance of factors other than hormonal ones is explained to her. She should then be offered help which she can accept if she feels she needs it. It may be that the marriage guidance counsellor will be of more use to her than the progesterone.

Vaginal Secretions

The vagina depends for its physiological function upon lubrication with a secretion of mucus. This is maximal during sexual excitement but is also present at other times. The amount will vary from one woman to another and in the same woman at different times. It may vary with the menstrual cycle. Some women find it is increased in hot weather. It is less in women approaching the menopause. It is always a clear, sticky mucus, not purulent or milky. It causes no discomfort, soreness or irritation. When stale it may have a strong odour which worries some women. Most women discover by experience what is a normal amount of vaginal secretion for them but sometimes one will be unnerved by a magazine article or friendly informant into thinking that what she has is a sign of disease. If she goes to the doctor telling him she has a vaginal discharge and if, as is common practice, he then gives her a prescription for pessaries, she never finds out she is normal and he, with little hope of success, treats a non-existent infection.

The vagina and vulva reflect a woman's well being as much as does her face and women who are tired, depressed or chronically unhappy may find the vagina dry and the vulva sore and uncomfortable. The mucosa may look dry and red and it is more likely to become infected.

At the same time as cultivating an awareness of the importance of the influence of stress on gynaecological symptoms, it is clearly necessary to continue to be watchful for symptoms of diagnosable and treatable disease.

A certain amount of vulval discomfort and soreness and vaginal discharge from time to time is the normal experience of all women and it is a great mistake to apply creams and pessaries in the absence of clear evidence of infection. This does not mean that every doctor working in general practice should always carry out a vaginal examination and high vaginal swab before he writes a prescription for pessaries. The diagnosis of a recurrence of vaginal thrush in a woman who has had it before and recognises the symptoms may reasonably be made on the history alone and treated without examination, provided that the doctor makes sure that there are no more sinister symptoms than itching and white discharge and the woman understands that she should return if her symptoms persist. However it is important that this does not become the standard practice for the management of all women who complain of vaginal discharge or vulval soreness. Not only is the doctor likely to miss the correct diagnosis but he may never know what the basis of the patient's anxiety really is. Her complaint of vaginal discharge may obscure a sexual problem, a fear of being not quite normal, of having venereal disease or cancer. She may have good reason for these fears or they may be imaginary. The doctor can neither treat the disease nor allay the anxieties if he does not make a diagnosis. To do this he must take a history and examine the patient. The history will reveal whether the complaint represents a change in the woman's usual state or only a change in her attitude to it.

It is important to ask specifically whether there has been any intermenstrual, post-coital or post-menopausal bleeding even if these were not the original complaint. The patient will not necessarily recognise the most important symptoms, or if she does, may be afraid to mention them. It is useful to know the character of the discharge, whether it is continuous or intermittent, how long ago it started and whether it is accompanied by any other symptom such as pain, irritation, dyspareunia, frequency or dysuria. The method of contraception used may also be relevant.

Examination

The doctor should not expect every woman to tell him the extent of her sexual activities but he should make it clear to her that if there is a possibility of venereal disease, then she should go to a special clinic. A statement to this effect relieves her of the necessity of answering if she does not want to and at the same time impresses on her that it is not possible to exclude venereal disease in general practice but requires special facilities. If necessary he should explain what venereal disease is and how it is contracted.

The abdomen should always be examined first, partly because it may reveal a surprise like a pregnancy or tumour and partly because it is then easier to proceed to a vaginal examination. A good light and speculum are essential. Lubricants and antiseptics must not be used if a smear or high vaginal swab is to be taken. The vulva should be inspected first. Vulval warts are common and often associated with discharge and irritation and often unnoticed by the patient. Although very rare in practice, it would be a pity to miss a primary chancre. In the elderly, it is important to look for leukoplakia. A urethral caruncle may cause soreness and dysuria. The advantage of carrying out many vaginal examinations on normal women is that the doctor becomes familiar with the normal appearance. The abnormal is then easier to recognise. In thrush, the vagina is bright red, the so-called 'raw beef' appearance, and there is a curdy white discharge. In trichomonas or mixed infections, the mucosa is purplish and the discharge yellow and profuse. A high vaginal swab should be taken. A swab of discharge from the vulva is useless. Charcoal swabs should be taken from the cervical os and the urethra and placed in a transport medium as it is sometimes possible to identify gonorrhoea from these, although immediate examination and culture of the swabs, such as is carried out in venereal disease clinics, yields a much higher success rate.

A cervical smear should be taken and may contribute to the diagnosis in infection. It may have to be repeated if there is severe cervicitis because of the difficulty of interpretation of the result. A bimanual examination must be done when there is a complaint of vaginal discharge, dyspareunia, low abdominal or back pain as an accurate diagnosis of salpingitis or even a suspicion of an early tubal pregnancy may be possible.

Management of Gynaecological Problems

There are many preparations of creams and pessaries available for the treatment of vaginal infections. There does not seem much to choose between them. The doctor has to make up his own mind which one to prescribe, bearing in mind any preference the patient may have and the likelihood of monilial infection. If a trichomonas infection is confirmed then a course of oral metronidazole is the best treatment for both the woman and her male partner. Recurrent infection with monilia sometimes responds to a course of oral nystatin or amphotericin B. It may be useful to tell the patient some of the factors which make women more likely to develop thrush so that they can try to avoid them. These include hot climates and surroundings, especially hot baths and several layers of nylon clothing, soap, bath salts, antibiotics and the oral contraceptive pill. Vinegar or salt in the bath may be helpful. Women subject to thrush are to be advised to avoid unnecessary courses of antibiotics even more than other people. They may find it helpful to stop the pill for three months while the condition is treated. If pelvic infection develops with an intra-uterine contraceptive device in place, it should be removed.

If a woman on the pill is found to have a severe cervical erosion it is usually necessary to stop the pill to allow it to heal. It may then be possible for her to take it again but she should be examined again after three months and again after a further six months to check that it has not recurred. If it keeps recurring it may be better for her to try a different method of contraception. If she is very anxious to continue in the first instance, and if the smear is reported as no worse than Class 2, it is worth trying a course of pessaries like hydrargaphen or to treat any definite infection and examine her again in three months.

Many women complaining of vulval discomfort or pelvic pain have an underlying sexual problem. This will be discussed in Chapter 4.

Women with the following conditions should be referred to a gynaecologist:

1. Post-menopausal bleeding, unless it is clearly due to senile vaginitis, cervical and posterior fornix smears are satisfactory and it responds quickly to local hormones.
2. Intermenstrual or post-coital bleeding for which no cause (e.g. erosion) is found or which fails to respond to treatment.
3. A smear reported as Class 3 or worse on two successive occasions.
4. A severe erosion even if the smear is reported as Class 2.
5. Ovarian swellings other than small cysts.
6. Leukoplakia.
7. Cervical polyps.

If there is a serious likelihood of venereal infection, and the woman refuses to attend a venereal disease clinic, then the general practitioner must investigate with swabs and serology and treat as best he can, recognising the limitations imposed on him.

There is no clear evidence that routine screening with cervical smears of all healthy women has any beneficial results. However, many women now believe it to be necessary and important, and most doctors will agree to do one if requested. The biggest problem is whether, and if so how often, women should be recommended to have cervical smears. There is no logical reason for carrying them out more often in women on the pill than others, which is what is usually done at present.

There is some sense in doing a smear whenever a woman is having a vaginal examination for another reason, for instance a post-natal examination, before starting the pill or because she has a symptom. Apart from this, certain women are particularly at risk from carcinoma of the cervix and it is reasonable to examine them regularly. They include those who have had a precociously early start to their sex life, those who have had many consorts and those who have had four or more pregnancies. Women with husbands in dirty occupations also seem to be particularly at risk. It is least likely to be found in virgins and in women from social classes 1 or 2 with one husband and few or no children.

4 LOVE AND SEX

'Love is the contact of two skins.' From the moment of birth, mother and child share a need for and a pleasure in close physical contact. It is initially a purely sensual pleasure but it forms the basis of lifelong binding affection which expands to include intellectual as well as emotional love.

Mature sexual love is a combination of this basic sexually undifferentiated love with sexual drive. It is the mutual reflection of physical, emotional and intellectual needs. How man developed this unique background to a method of reproduction, which in other respects is similar to other mammals, is not clear. One explanation is that it was a biological necessity based on natural selection, while some people look on it as a manifestation of man's God-given spirituality. For whatever reason, successful human sexual relationships require elements of physical, emotional and intellectual love and interdependence. The ability to make such a relationship depends on experience in infancy. Just as someone who does not hear speech in early childhood never becomes fully fluent and articulate, those who are deprived of early mothering, including close physical contact, fail to develop the capacity for successful sexual relationships in adult life. If the child's relationship with the mother or mother substitute is delayed by early separation or interrupted during early life, the child's capacity for successful relationships is permanently damaged. Some overcome the handicap to a certain extent but the effect is never completely lost.

Sexual Conditioning in Children

As well as a capacity for love, adults need a knowledge and understanding of sexuality and sexual technique. How they gain this and what they learn will influence their sexual behaviour. Attitudes to sex are learned at an early age from parents and later from the peer group, teachers and the media. If parents openly delight in physical contact with each other and with their children and are relaxed about nudity, the child learns at an early age the sensual pleasure of the contact of two skins as well as the anatomical difference between the sexes. The knowledge is absorbed along with numerous other items of information and forms the practical base for the theoretical facts about human reproduction which she will learn later. The earliest impressions are

Love and Sex

formed in a totally innocent mind, free from any ideas of shame, secrecy or moral judgement. The infant's pleasure in playing with the nipple, masturbation or defaecation is blatant and unashamed. Any modification of this behaviour has to be learned.

If the parents are able to treat sex in a relaxed way and teach the child that it is enjoyable though private she will grow up without disabling inhibitions. If their own attitude to sensual pleasure, from physical contact and nudity to sexual intercourse, is one of guilt and repression, then she will grow up believing it to be a necessary evil to be ashamed of and regretted rather than rejoiced in. If, when she is young, she forms the impression that sex is dirty and disgusting she is unlikely ever to be able to welcome and enjoy it.

In order to develop the capacity for happy heterosexual relationships in adult life, children of both sexes need to observe love and mutual respect between their parents. If the father is a violent or aggressive man of whom the mother or children are afraid, the girls grow up to look on sex as an expression of violence and aggression and to be fearful of it. The boys fail to develop the ability to view women with gentleness and respect and a sexual relationship as an expression of love and shared pleasure.

Early conditioning is among the commonest causes of frigidity in women. There is now widespread support in the media for the sexual emancipation of women, but the inhibiting attitudes which are implanted early in the young infant are too powerful and too firmly rooted to be ousted by later influences. In fact the widespread publicity about what she should be experiencing often contrasts so sharply with what a woman is in fact experiencing that it increases her anxiety and guilt and therefore her problems.

During her early life, as well as forming attitudes to sexuality, the child learns about sexual roles within the family. She will observe her parents behaviour towards each other and towards herself and any other children. Her model for herself as wife and mother will be based on what she observes as a child. Problems may arise if this model conflicts with ideas such as career ambitions which she develops later or with the expectations which her husband brings to the marriage based on his own early observations.

If a girl's mother is a domesticated, maternal woman and her parent's relationship a traditional one with her father going out to work and contributing little to the running of the home while her mother enjoys and takes pride in caring for her husband and children and being responsible for the domestic organisation, she may find it difficult herself to combine marriage and a career. Even if her husband is happy and willing to share the domestic chores, she may feel guilty that she is not fulfilling her wifely role. If she gives up the career, she feels frustrated and resentful.

Conversely, she may be quite happy to accept the sharing of the running of the household with her husband but he is unable to forget his early wife-model in the form of his mother, who was devoted and caring and the servant of his father and himself. Intellectually, he wants his wife to be happy and fulfilled. Emotionally, he resents that she is not a proper wife to him and that he has to do women's work helping her in the house. Such conflicts may have repercussions on the couple's sex life which they may be unable to resolve without professional help.

Sexual Problems

There are few people who do not have sexual difficulties at some time during their lives. Most are not serious or persistent, and most do not need help from a doctor or anyone else. However, a large number of the patients attending the surgery are unhappy about their sex lives, even if they do not ask for help in this respect. Many of these become anxious and develop neurotic symptoms. Their health quotient deteriorates and they become vulnerable to illness, both organic and emotional. It is a waste of time treating the symptoms without at least recognising the underlying cause or contributing factor. It is therefore necessary for members of the health team to be aware of the range of sexual problems and their importance if they are to be fully equipped to deal with all aspects of clinical practice.

The extent to which a general practitioner can treat sexual problems will be limited by his knowledge and understanding and by his interest and skill in psychotherapy and in developing the techniques necessary for the more difficult cases. This means that he will generally be able to do something for the vast majority, who need information and reassurance and help in recognising and accepting the problem, but will be unlikely to be able to treat successfully the small group with serious difficulties. It is doubtful whether anything can be done to help this group as specialised treatment is available on such a small scale as to be unattainable for most. Even when it is available, the problems are often so much a part of the subject's personality as to be resistant to treatment. As with other disabilities, even when they cannot be cured, the primary health care team has an important part to play in helping people to learn to live with them and minimise their effects. If people can openly discuss their difficulties with someone who will not be

Love and Sex 49

shocked or censorious, then they may be prevented from having wider repercussions on their health and relationships.

Occasionally a sexual problem is important in its own right and in isolation from other aspects of the patient's life. More often it is associated with other difficulties. Not only are people who are happy, mature and well adjusted less likely to have a sexual problem in the first place but they are also better equipped to sort it out on their own if they do.

Most of the sexual problems met by the primary health care team will be among the following two groups:

Clinical (i.e. Individual Cases)

Parental anxiety about masturbation and sex-play in children.
Problems of sexual identity, ignorance and fear in the young.
Marital problems: non-consummation, impotence, premature ejaculation, vaginismus, frigidity and failure to achieve orgasm in women.
Infertility.
Contraception.
Venereal disease.
Miscellaneous: indecent exposure, transvestism, homosexual problems, sexual crimes.

Social

Attitudes: within the primary health care team, within schools, within the rest of the community.
Education: of children by parents, of children in school, of parents and teachers, of other adults.

Both doctors and patients often have difficulty in discussing sex in detail and this can lead to a great deal of wasted time. The patient may feel obliged to come to the doctor with another complaint, only telling him about the real problem if she finds him sympathetic. Even then, if she senses he is embarrassed, she may approach the subject in a roundabout way.

It is impossible to take a full medical history without including sexual performance among the other bodily functions. This is particularly important when the patient is obviously suffering from a psychiatric illness, but also relevant in a wide range of other conditions including all the stress-related diseases such as asthma, peptic ulcer and hypertension. A doctor who finds it difficult to discuss sex may be able to desensitise himself to the subject by introducing it more often with patients, among colleagues or at home. He should be able to approach it with the same ease as micturition or bowel function. Even if a doctor has no interest in sexual problems and does not intend to treat them himself, he must be capable of identifying them in his patients so that he can refer them to someone else.

As well as being approachable and at ease when discussing sex, the professional worker has to be able to recognise and discard his own prejudices. To start with he must have a clear idea of what constitutes a sexual problem. Human sexual behaviour is varied and a patient does not have a problem just because the doctor finds what she does distasteful or even immoral. It may be of importance if the patient considers it immoral, but that is another matter. A sexual problem exists if the subject or her partner, if she has one, finds her sex life unsatisfactory and her sexual tensions unrelieved. She does not have a problem just because her performance fails to match up to some external standard quoted in a magazine or because the doctor thinks her behaviour unnatural. An unconsummated marriage is not a problem if the couple are happy and well and fulfilled and do not want children. This may be unusual but the subject must be approached with an open mind which allows the possibility.

It is essential to establish first whether there really is a problem, i.e. is the patient or the couple unhappy or dissatisfied or are they simply anxious that what they are doing is unnatural, harmful or failing to measure up to some mythical norm? Many people lack the self-confidence to continue to do what pleases them without official recognition that it is satisfactory. It should take only a few moments to discover whether what the patient is presenting is a true problem or not. The only other important point is to discover whether or not a couple want to conceive and to confirm that their sexual behaviour is compatible with their wishes in this respect. If they indulge only in oral sex or masturbation or intercourse only during menstruation, they clearly will not conceive, even if they want to, whereas if they are having normal sexual intercourse without using contraceptives they probably will, even if they do not want to.

Taking the History

Having established that there is a true sexual problem, it will be necessary to enquire further into the patient's history. A standard pattern of questions is useful but it may not elicit some of the most important information relating to the problem itself. If the doctor or counsellor is alert he may find the patient ready to expand, if given the chance, while

Love and Sex 51

answering the more mundane questions.

History of Present Complaint

Nature of the problem as exactly as possible.
Duration/frequency: when did it start? — did this follow some event, e.g. confinement, moving house? — is it always present or only sometimes? — has it happened in the past and been resolved? — is it the same under all circumstances, e.g. on holiday, Sunday afternoons, with a different partner, when the children are away?
Effect of the problem: on well being, marriage.
Bodily functions: appetite, sleep, bowels, micturition.

Previous History — Medical and Sexual

Illnesses, operations, pregnancies and their relationship, if any, to the problem.
Psychiatric illness.
Sexual learning and experience: in childhood — in adolescence — in earlier adult life — early learning, traumatic experiences, pre- and extramarital experience. Attitudes to opposite sex and to own sex.

Family History

Relationships within family: parents with each other — parents with children — children with each other.
Family attitudes to sex.
Are parents and siblings alive and well now?

Personal History

Occupation: hours, quality, satisfaction, pay.
Finances: how is family money organised — does wife know what husband earns? — who decides how it is spent?
Marriage: relationship, shared interests, separate interests. Points of conflict — frequency and violence of conflict.
Children: ages, sexes, attitudes to them, anxieties about them, relationships between them.
Contraception: method, attitude, degree of satisfaction with method. Any conflict over it?
Anxieties, fears, attitudes.
Drinking habits.
Smoking habits.

This sounds very time-consuming and detailed but most of it can usually be skipped through quite quickly. At the end of it, many of the problems will obviously be virtually non-existent, or transitory and associated with some minor domestic upset. Talking about it will have helped and nothing more be needed. But a few clearly need further attention.

Sexual problems are often blamed on physical disease, and almost every known condition has been implicated, but the connection is most often due to coincidence or to secondary effects of illness such as depression and financial problems. However, it is sensible to test urine for sugar in women with vaginal thrush and in impotent men. Apart from this it is probably only necessary to examine people with the following: symptoms suggestive of physical abnormality or disease, fear of physical abnormality or disease, dyspareunia, vaginal or urethral discharge.

Sexuality in Children

Parents often worry about evidence of sexuality in children. Only a few ever express their anxiety and it would probably be helpful if more were encouraged to do so. A skilful health visitor should be able to give every mother an opportunity to talk about her anxieties. Some will be worried about how to tell their children about sex. Some girls still start menstruation knowing nothing about it. Discussion with the health visitor may remove some of the woman's embarrassment, improve her own knowledge and vocabulary and enable her to talk freely with her children.

Masturbation is a common parental worry. Most people now accept that it is harmless if it is not done 'too much' but even doctors cannot agree on where the dividing line should be drawn or what the dangers are. In fact there is no evidence whatsoever that it is ever harmful although it may be a symptom of insecurity or unhappiness — a sort of comfort habit.

Parents may visit the doctor with the sole purpose of discussing masturbation. Others will come with vague anxieties about the child's health or saying that she has a sore vulva, nocturnal enuresis or difficulty or pain on passing urine. No help can be given unless the real nature of their anxiety can be brought out into the open. The doctor or health visitor must help by asking whether the child masturbates, if necessary explaining what this means, and if so, asking whether this worries them.

Usually discussion and reassurance is all that is needed. If the parents can accept that masturbation is universal and harmless they should be able to stop worrying. If it seems as though the parents are particularly

Love and Sex

upset about what they see as a serious problem or perversion, and are likely to punish the child, the dangers of such actions need to be explained to them. It is clear that punishing masturbation, or even being excessively censorious about it, can produce sexual problems in adolescence or adult life. The most that parents should do is to make it clear that public sex in any form is socially unacceptable.

It may be helpful to discover and to help them to understand why they are so worried about the matter. Their fears may be based on childhood experience or on anxiety that the child will be sexually precocious. They may find the doctor's bland reassurance difficult to accept. Some may be persuaded by reading a book on the subject, and others, even if they cannot read well enough, may be reassured by the knowledge that there are books which support what the doctor is saying.

Similar anxieties arise about sex-play between young children. This arises more from curiosity than the gratification of sexual impulses and is as harmless as masturbation unless the parents over-react. Parents' reaction can result in the ostracism of a child who has been blamed for initiating sex-play in a local community. This not only has a disastrous effect on the victim but also makes all the other children involved wary and secretive about sex. The parents are in effect telling all the children that it is bad, dirty, wrong. Some will grow to fear it. Some will develop an unhealthy interest in it at an early age.

Sexual Development in Adolescence

Adolescence is an unsettled, even stormy time for many people. Sexual development is the most obvious change taking place and is often bewildering even to the most well-informed youngster. However much she knows about the facts of sex, nobody can tell her what she will feel like at this time. It is difficult to describe the emotional turmoil and sense of isolation many adolescents experience. To each one it is uniquely difficult, often mystifying, sometimes frightening. Their most urgent need is to talk about their feelings and fears. Once given expression, they lose their immense significance and can be faced. If they remain unspoken they can grow and expand to terrifying proportions.

Few young people feel able to talk to their parents about these problems. This is not necessarily evidence of a breakdown in family relationships. Even if these are good, parents are too close, too much involved, too caring to be able to share such agonising confidences. The feelings the adolescent needs to describe are part fantasy, part unfounded fears, which she is likely to recognise as such, while still feeling anxious about them. She knows that her parents can only dismiss them as ridiculous. At the same time they would feel worried by what are sometimes apparently bizarre revelations and hurt by those aspects of them which involve themselves. What is needed is a sensible, uninvolved counsellor, capable of recognising serious problems needing more specialised help, who will listen and comfort and where possible reassure the girl that she is normal. Such a person can be instrumental in preventing serious emotional disturbance, promiscuity or delinquency. Who will play this role will depend on whom the girl feels she can most easily turn to and trust. It may be a relation, neighbour or teacher, or it may be a member of the primary health care team. If there is no one, or the chosen person rejects her and she cannot resolve her difficulties, then she may try to draw comfort from alcohol, drugs or a too intense sexual relationship. She may become pregnant, commit crimes or attempt suicide, all ways of drawing attention to what she finds an intolerable situation.

The commonest sexually based anxieties of adolescents involve fantasies about relationships with people of either sex, not necessarily known to them, fears of being abnormal, unattractive or incapable of normal sex, fears of pregnancy or venereal disease, unease about their own sexual orientation and fears of homosexuality. A number of the boys will indulge in private transvestism or indecent exposure. Many will need factual information and contraceptive advice.

The Sexual Problems of Couples

The vast majority of sexual problems brought to a general practitioner are those of married couples. Most often, one member of the couple comes and insists that the other is not included in any discussion. Many women feel that the problem, for instance failure to achieve orgasm, is theirs alone. Many couples never discuss sex — some never discuss anything — and the suggestion that they should do so alarms them. They may consider it quite impossible. Nevertheless, every attempt should be made to include both partners as no marital sexual problem involves exclusively one or other. It must be treated as a failure, if that is what it is, of the couple as a unit.

Non-problems are common and must not be dismissed too quickly. The patient should be given time to explain what is worrying her and why, if she is to accept the advice that it is not important.

The idea that they are not as sexually active as they used to be, or as other couples are, is a common source of anxiety. Some couples worry that they are still enjoying sex at an age when they think perhaps they should not, others that they find particular times of day, situations or

Love and Sex

positions most pleasurable. For some, if normal sex has become impossible due to age or disease, for instance after vulvectomy or prostatectomy, they may worry about the pleasure they find in mutual masturbation. All these should be reassured that what they are doing is normal, healthy, safe, and common practice.

It is self-evident that a man needs to be sexually aroused and to have an erect penis before intercourse can take place. It is less obvious that for her to enjoy sexual intercourse, the woman also must be at an advanced stage of arousal before penetration is attempted. This means that the whole vulva should be congested and swollen (or 'erect') and well lubricated with mucus. If penetration is attempted before this stage is reached, it may be painful and cause vaginismus, either then or at later attempts; it may cause cystitis and the woman is unlikely to reach orgasm before the man's is finished. The most sensitive parts of the woman being more closely hidden than the man's, she may not be aroused by sexual foreplay which is not specifically and deliberately directed to those areas. Her husband should be prepared to stimulate her before penetration in whatever way she finds most pleasurable and she should be prepared to guide him in this.

The degree of sex drive or libido varies between individuals and in individuals at different times in their lives. It is therefore likely that partners will find their needs at variance, at least at certain times. It is widely believed that men have a higher level of libido than women but this is by no means always the case and some wives would like more frequent intercourse than their husbands can manage. An important difference is that whereas a woman can submit to sex to please her husband even if she does not desire it, he cannot do the same for her.

It is said that most men reach their maximum sexuality during their early twenties, while for women the peak is five to ten years later. In addition to this a woman's libido is more easily reduced by fatigue and anxiety and is especially likely to be low for a year after a confinement. For these reasons, and possibly as a result of social conditioning and physiological differences, women are more usually satisfied with a lower frequency of sexual intercourse than men. Within marriage, both partners may have to modify their demands and most couples arrive at a mutually acceptable level of intercourse, with perhaps occasional masturbation if one feels dissatisfied.

Some may need help in coming to a compromise solution and in understanding and accepting that they are both normal: that the man is not a sex maniac because he would like intercourse every night (unless of course he insists on it) nor the woman frigid and unloving because she really cannot face it more often than twice a week. It may be that the woman will in fact become more enthusiastic about sex if she is helped not to feel guilty about her reluctance, nor pressured into what is for her too frequent intercourse. If her anxiety can be reduced, then she may achieve an orgasm more easily and her libido may in fact increase. She should try to understand how hurt her husband feels when, in addition to being too busy with the new baby to pay much attention to him, she also rejects his sexual advances. He should understand that her behaviour is normal for a woman with a baby and does not mean she has stopped loving him. They can both be reassured that, if they are patient and loving and have shared a mutually enjoyable sex life in the past, it will return.

Loss of libido in women is the commonest sexual problem. Sexual enthusiasm in a woman and the ease with which she can be aroused is a much more fragile thing than in her male partner. Even during lovemaking it can evaporate as a result of a sound from a child, an irrelevant thought or a tactless word from her partner. Most women find it difficult to be sexually interested after an unresolved argument or during a more prolonged period of chronic disagreement. A reduced interest in sex may be one of the earliest symptoms of anxiety or depression. If one of these conditions becomes chronic she may lose all enthusiasm for lovemaking. Her attitude in itself will cause stresses within the marriage and unless both partners understand how it has arisen the problem may become self-perpetuating.

The role of any counsellor must be to help the couple to understand what is happening to them and why and to find their own way towards a solution.

The problems of the couple who have never achieved a sexual relationship satisfactory to both partners are much more difficult. The likelihood of them resolving the problem spontaneously is less the longer they continue. The commonest difficulty is that the woman fails to reach her orgasm by the time the man's is over. This may be because he suffers from premature ejaculation and his orgasm occurs soon after or even before penetration. Alternatively it may be that she is particularly slow to reach orgasm.

Premature ejaculation is said to respond to the squeeze technique in which the woman squeezes the penis at the level of the corona between the thumb and first two fingers, the thumb being placed beneath the penis and the fingers above. She does this as soon as ejaculation seems imminent and continues the pressure until the sensation has worn off. The process is repeated and enables the man to maintain an erection for longer.

Love and Sex

It can help for foreplay between the partners to be focused more on the woman with manual stimulation of the clitoris or vulval area in general in whatever way she finds most exciting. If penetration is delayed until she has progressed a considerable way towards full arousal then she is more likely to achieve orgasm at the same time as, or before, her husband.

A continuing interest in sexual technique and willingness to experiment can be major factors in avoiding the sexual boredom which sometimes affects marriages of long-standing which are in other respects satisfactory.

No woman will find full satisfaction from intercourse if it is painful. Dyspareunia can be caused by local disease of the vulva, vagina or pelvic organs, by dryness due to hormonal deficiency, to vaginismus due to emotional problems or to poor sexual technique. It is important to examine all women with this complaint and to take a high vaginal swab. If there seems to be no structural reason for the complaint, the other possibilities should be considered. Vaginismus should be easy to diagnose as it is likely to make vaginal examination difficult or impossible and this forms a good opportunity to introduce the discussion. She is likely to have a deep-rooted fear of sex and it may help to talk about this. She should then be encouraged to examine herself in the bath or with a lubricant, starting by inserting the tip of one finger and then progressing to a whole finger and then two. She may then allow the tip of the erect penis to lie in the vulva if she holds it. It may help to experiment with different positions – lying on their sides facing each other or with the woman on top. She may then gradually be able to accept full intercourse. If she is unable to do so, or unable to achieve orgasm at all, or only with masturbation, and particularly if she finds sex altogether distasteful, then she may have deep-seated emotional problems which require skilled psychotherapy. If this is not available or there is a long waiting list, the GP or CPN may be able to help the couple to maintain a loving and understanding relationship in the meantime. Masturbation should not be frowned on or discouraged in this situation.

Sex After Surgery

Preparation of patients for surgery is usually very badly done. They are not told what the operation entails, what they will feel like afterwards, how long they will remain in hospital, whether they can expect to recover completely and if so how long it will take, let alone when it will be done or by whom.

It is well known among doctors that men are often impotent for a time after prostatectomy. If they are to recover they have to keep on trying. It is also well known that if a man has once found himself impotent, his confidence is shaken and he may be afraid to try again. Despite this, most men and their wives are not warned of the possibility before the operation. They are shattered by the discovery at their first attempt and never try again. The impotence becomes permanent.

Following hysterectomy, a woman may feel nervous of intercourse, be unable to respond to her husband's lovemaking and experience a reduction in natural lubrication and dyspareunia. Most of these symptoms rapidly disappear as long as they are expected, understood and treated patiently by both partners. They become permanent if they are not.

A lot of readjustment will have to be achieved by both partners if they are to continue a satisfying sex life after mastectomy. The woman feels that her husband cannot possibly love her any more and he may indeed be temporarily repulsed by her disfigurement.

The role of the members of the primary health care team in these situations is clear — to inform, comfort and reassure. If the vagina has been shortened or the vault is tender, it may help for the woman to keep her legs together during intercourse during the early post-operative weeks and only to experiment with full penetration gently at a later time.

A radical vulvectomy is a much more mutilating and sexually incapacitating operation. Both husband and wife should be seen before the operation and warned that they may not be able to resume normal intercourse afterwards. At least they then have a better chance of continuing a loving relationship within this limitation. If they are not warned, the discovery may come as a shock and they may become anxious and blame each other for their difficulties.

Sex in Old Age

Many women feel that they should not continue to have sexual intercourse after the menopause. Some want to and enjoy it and feel guilty. Some, usually those who have never found any great pleasure in it, are relieved to have an excuse not to continue. Men may be affected by their wives' feelings and made to feel guilty. There is clearly nothing intrinsically wrong in continuing regular intercourse into old age if both partners desire it. In fact when the couple have more time, fewer pressures and no need to worry about contraception, they may find a renewed pleasure in their relationship. Those couples most likely to continue a satisfactory sexual relationship into old age are those who found it most enjoyable when young and who did not allow it to lapse during their fifties when interest often wanes for a while.

In middle age and after, women may be particularly diffident about mentioning sexual anxieties to a doctor, especially a young man, and may hesitate to reveal that they still have sexual feelings at all. It is therefore more than ever desirable in this group for the doctor to introduce the subject if it seems likely that there may be anxiety underlying the presenting symptoms. He should in any case ask whether there has been bleeding between the periods or since menstruation ceased. He should in the same breath ask whether there is bleeding or pain associated with intercourse. The woman may answer by saying 'we don't do it any more' and the doctor can ask whether this is by choice or because of some problem. By asking the question in the first place, he has made it clear that it would be normal for her to be having regular sex. Even if no further conversation follows, her anxiety may be relieved.

If there is dyspareunia due to vaginal dryness or senile vaginitis then a lubricant or oestrogen cream may help.

If a woman has always found sex distasteful, then it is unlikely that she can be helped to start enjoying it after middle age but she may be persuaded to be tolerant towards her husband and not look upon him as a perverted beast because he still has sexual desires.

Sexual problems and the anxiety which surrounds them can both cause and be caused by a low health quotient. It is therefore important that the primary health care team takes them seriously and does its best to relieve them. Which member of the team is involved will vary according to the local situation and the preference of the patient, but the marriage guidance counsellor and the community psychiatric nurse are the most likely to be interested.

5 CONCEPTION AND CONTRACEPTION

Conception

This is the simplest of subjects for the primary health care team and yet gives rise to the most complicated situations. People coming to the surgery for help in this field have one of only two problems: either they do not want to conceive or they do and cannot. It is what follows from these simple problems which may be complex.

The infertile couple may need information only, complicated investigation, referral for surgery, artificial insemmination, medication or advice on adoption. Those who do not want to conceive need help in realising when they are at risk, and in choosing and using a method of contraception. They may also seek abortion or help in coping with an unplanned pregnancy.

The route to all these things lies through the primary health care team. Failure or inadequacy in their provision can lead to misery, morbidity and a lowered health quotient.

Many people of all ages are ignorant of how their bodies work. In some areas this may not be much of a problem but it can be of importance in the matter of conception: both how to achieve it and how to avoid it. It is important for the success of the management of infertility as well as the use of contraception for the patient to be as well informed as possible. This is not a form of treatment which can be used on the patient without her active co-operation and understanding. The doctor must listen and find out what the patient already knows so that he can reinforce what is correct and counter the mistakes. He should be prepared to draw diagrams of how conception occurs – both structural ones of the organs concerned and a chart of the physiological process of menstruation and ovulation. These must be intelligible to the patient so that she understands what lies behind any advice she receives and any investigations which may be undertaken.

Very often a woman will worry at not having conceived within a very short time of starting to try. The first visit can therefore be spent in ensuring that she has a normal menstrual history, understands conception, confirming that both she and her husband are fit and having regular normal intercourse during the fertile period, i.e. around 14 days before the next period is due, and without contraception. A vaginal examination should be done if she has not already had one. Most doctors would not want to go further than this for at least a year. The couple should then be seen together and warned that further tests may show that one or other is solely responsible for the problem and that this may cause stresses in their relationship for which they should be prepared. Then it is usual to do the simple things first — the seminal fluid should be examined and the woman asked to keep a chart of her early morning temperature. The sperm count should be repeated several times if it is low or borderline. The temperature chart should be kept for at least three months as it is unlikely to be kept accurately to start with, the usual pattern may be destroyed by a virus infection, hangover or forgetfulness and it is impossible to see a regular repeating pattern in fewer than three cycles. Ovulation is usually indicated by a rise in temperature. It may be shown to be occurring at an unusual time in the cycle and intercourse can then be timed to coincide with ovulation.

If conception still has not occurred and both partners ask for further investigation, the couple should be referred to a unit with a special interest in the problem. They should be warned before they go that they may not always understand fully what is happening at the hospital and should be encouraged to return to the GP for elucidation if necessary.

Contraception

A woman asking for contraceptive advice before starting a family should be asked whether she has had rubella vaccination. If not she may be offered it at this stage, if she can be trusted not to become pregnant during the next three months, or a blood test for rubella antibodies may be done. If it is negative she should be warned that she should have the vaccine before starting a pregnancy.

Contraception is needed by all sexually active women of childbearing age having heterosexual relationships. Properly used, it should enable most women to avoid unplanned pregnancies. It is of the utmost importance that information about contraception is easily available, accurate and detailed. The primary health care team and the family planning clinics are the only reliable sources of information and more women are turning to their GP than ever before. This aspect of the GP's work has hitherto been decidedly amateurish in many instances. Now that doctors are paid by the FPC for providing contraceptive advice there is no excuse, if ever there was one, for it to be less than first class.

The first task is to determine whether there are any special factors which render a particular method more or less suitable for any individual woman. It is then useful to discover what she already knows about contraception and whether she herself favours a particular method. If she does, then this is the one most likely to succeed.

The Pill

The oral contraceptive in the form of a pill combining an oestrogen and a progestogen is the commonest method now in use and certainly the most reliable. It carries minimal risks for a young, non-smoker with normal blood pressure and is the method of choice for most women under thirty-five. The dose of oestrogen should not be greater than 30 mcg. The dose of progestogen depends upon which preparation is used.

Although there has been talk of making the pill generally available, there are advantages to retaining the present system whereby it can be obtained only on prescription. This means that the doctor carries the responsibility, as when prescribing any drug, of making sure it is taken only by women for whom it is safe, who understand how to use it and who receive regular checks. The patient of course retains the responsibility of making sure she understands the doctor's instructions, follows them and makes her own practical and moral decisions about whether and when to have sex. The main advantages of oral contraception with the combined pill are that it is easy and convenient to use, provides a high degree of contraceptive reliability, regulates the menstrual cycle and diminishes menstrual loss and pain. The disadvantages of the pill are that it carries risks for certain people, not all of whom can be identified beforehand, has minor side-effects for some people and interferes with the body's normal physiological processes.

Before prescribing the pill, a full history should be taken to assess the importance of contraception and particularly pill contraception to this woman and to discover any contra-indications. Most of the contra-indications to taking the pill are relative. That is, there may be circumstances in which the pill may be the only alternative to pregnancy in a woman for whom it may carry risks, but for whom pregnancy would be disastrous and who cannot use any other method. On the whole it should not be taken by women who:

— do not have a regular cycle established for at least a year
— have scanty and irregular periods and whose family is not complete
— have recently had hepatitis or whose liver-function tests remain grossly abnormal after an earlier attack of hepatitis
— have a history of pulmonary embolism, deep-vein thrombosis or cerebral thrombosis or myocardial infarction
— have had carcinoma of breast or genital tract
— have hypertension-diastolic persistently over 90
— are over 35 and smoke

Conception and Contraception 63

— are over 40
— are awaiting surgery
— are taking drugs known to antagonise the pill (e.g. barbiturates, rifampicin).
It is not the method of choice in women with diabetes, bad varicose veins, a history of severe migraine, depression, epilepsy or sickle cell disease.

A combination of risk factors may amount to a more definite contraindication than a single one. For instance a heavy smoker of thirty-two with a bad family history of thromboembolic disease and mild essential hypertension probably should not take the pill. On the other hand, if a woman's life has been in a complete mess and all hope for the future depends upon satisfactory contraception during the next few months, a slightly higher risk may be acceptable than for another woman in quite different circumstances.

The doctor has to be prepared to explain these factors to the patient so that she may share in the decision-making.

The initial examination of a patient before starting to take the pill should include: weight, blood pressure, breasts, abdomen, legs for varicose veins, VE and cervical smear, and urine test.

Breast lumps should be investigated before starting the pill as must abdominal or pelvic swellings. If the blood pressure is raised at this first visit it should be repeated at least twice before a decision is made about the advisability of oral contraception.

Instructions to Patients Starting the Pill. (If sheath and pessaries are also being recommended instructions should be given for these too.)

1. Start taking it on the fifth day of the next period counting the day when bleeding starts as the first day, e.g. if the period starts on Monday, that is Day 1 then the first pill should be taken on Friday which is Day 5. It must be started on that day whether or not the period has finished. (Demonstrate with sample packet.)

2. Take one pill every day until the packet is finished.

3. Take the pill at about the same time every day — most women prefer bedtime.

4. If you forget to take it one day, i.e. it is still there when you go to take the next one, you are not protected for the rest of the month and must take no risks, i.e. not have intercourse or must use other precautions until after the next period.

5. If you have a stomach upset with diarrhoea or vomiting, the pill may not be properly absorbed. You may sick it up or it may go straight

through you without your knowing. Then you are in the same situation as if you had missed a pill and are not safe for the rest of the month.

6. If you forget to take the pill at the right time but remember within the next twelve hours, take it then and you are safe.

7. You are not safe until you have been taking the pill for two weeks. You should take other precautions or have no intercourse during that time.

8. The most suitable form of other precautions is usually for the man to use a sheath and the woman a spermicidal compound.

9. At the end of each packet, you have seven pill-free days i.e. you stop taking it for one week.

10. Then start the next packet.

11. You will probably have a period during the week you are not taking the pill. Do not worry if it doesn't come. Start taking the pill again at the right time anyway.

12. I am giving you a prescription for three packets now. Make an appointment to see me soon after you open the third packet so that you can tell me how you are getting on and collect a prescription for a further supply.

When she attends for the first follow-up visit she should be allowed time for general comments and then enquiry should be made as to whether she is taking the pill correctly. She should be asked specifically whether she has had periods during the pill-free weeks and whether there has been any bleeding while taking the pill. If all is well and her blood pressure is normal then she may be given a prescription for a further period. This is a good opportunity for pointing out that she may miss the pill-free week occasionally, taking it continuously for six weeks at a time if she wants to avoid having a period at a particular time.

If she has had no periods during the pill-free weeks it is important to check that she took no risks when starting the pill and has missed none. A pregnancy test should be done in any case. If pregnancy can be certainly excluded then she can continue to take the pill and ignore the amenorrhoea or she may try a preparation containing a higher dosage of progestogen.

Breakthrough bleeding during the first few cycles is common and if the initial examination was satisfactory need only be investigated if it persists.

Follow-up visits are usually at six-monthly intervals and along the same lines as the second visit. They can be carried out by a nurse. There is no reason why cervical smears should be done any more often in

Conception and Contraception 65

women on the pill than any other group. Every two to three years is usual.

The Sheath

The sheath is the second most popular method of contraception after the pill. It has had a reputation for unreliability but this is probably not justified when it is properly used. Like the pill, it needs to be issued with clear and detailed instructions, preferably both verbal and written. If these are provided, fully understood and followed then it can be a reasonably reliable method.

The advantages of the sheath are that it does not interfere with the body's normal physiology, that it can be used at short notice without the advance planning needed for other methods, and that it protects against venereal diseases and possibly carcinoma of the cervix.

The disadvantages are that lovemaking has to be interrupted for it to be applied with consequent loss of impetus for both partners, that it forms a barrier between the partners with diminished pleasurable sensation for both and that the man has to be entrusted with its use.

Instructions for Using a Sheath.

1. It must be used on every occasion that sexual intercourse takes place.

2. It is not a safe method unless the woman uses a spermicidal compound at the same time. This may be in the form of pessaries used with or without an applicator, cream, foam or gel used with an applicator.

3. The sheath can be applied only to an erect penis and care must be taken that there is no close contact between penis and the introitus before the sheath is on or after intercourse when it has been removed.

4. The penis must be removed from the vagina while still at least partially erect and the sheath must be held at the base of the penis as it is removed so that none of the seminal fluid leaks out.

The Cap

The most commonly used cap is in fact a vaginal diaphragm consisting of a domed sheet of thin rubber with a circular, coiled or flat spring around its base. It fits between the back of the pubic symphisis and the posterior fornix. Other types of cap which fit over the cervix itself are now rarely used.

The junction between the rim of the cap and the vaginal walls is not totally occlusive and the method works well only if a spermicidal compound is liberally applied in the cap and around its edge before it is inserted. If it is properly fitted and used it is a very good method. The diaphragm has to be fitted by someone who regularly does this work and is not out of practice. The woman should be shown how to use it and she should be examined after putting it in herself several times to make sure she is doing it correctly.

Inserting a cap correctly is quite difficult for some women and it is possible to position it between the pubic symphysis and the cervix, i.e. in the anterior fornix so that the cervix protrudes behind the cap – a most vulnerable position. The diaphragm may not fit properly if the woman gains or loses weight, is constipated or has a baby. The fit should be checked if any of these things happen and in any case once a year. It should be replaced about every six months. It should really be used every night even if intercourse seems unlikely. There is a great temptation not to do this and many women have taken risks because they did not feel like getting up later to insert the cap when it was in fact needed.

For all these reasons it is not a very popular method but it has advantages over the sheath and may be very useful for women who should not or do not wish to take the pill. These advantages are that it is inserted before lovemaking starts and therefore causes no interruption; if it fits properly, the couple should be unaware of its presence during intercourse; it has no effect on the body; it is extremely reliable and the responsibility for using it lies with the woman.

The IUCD

An intra-uterine contraceptive device consists of a piece of material, usually stiff plastic, coiled, folded or shaped in such a way that it can be inserted easily into the uterine cavity and which then remains there. Some of the devices are impregnated with progesterone or have fine copper wire coiled around the plastic. It is not clear exactly how the method works but it seems that the device irritates the lining of the uterus and causes a chronic inflammatory process which may discourage implantation of the ovum.

An IUCD does not in fact prevent conception, so from the point of view of the purist it is less a contraceptive device than an abortifacient. It clearly has a place for women who do not wish to use other methods and for whom it is suitable, but its disadvantages are great.

It causes an increase in the menstrual loss and for this reason should not be fitted in women who previously suffered from menorrhagia. In some women it causes endometritis with lower abdominal pain and irregular bleeding. Salpingitis and pyosalpinx are more common in women with IUCDs. Pregnancy occurs more frequently than with other contraceptive methods and if it does is more likely to be extra-uterine. Spontaneous abortion is common. There is some evidence that foetal abnormalities are more common in pregnancies which continue with an IUCD in place.

There are some women who experience none of these problems and for whom the method is suitable, but apart from excluding those with a previous history of menorrhagia or pelvic inflammatory disease, it is difficult to know which women are likely to have problems and which are not.

Sterilisation

Men. Vasectomy is a safe and simple operation, quick to perform under local anaesthetic and relatively free from complications or side-effects. It is most appropriate for the mature couple whose family is complete, but may sometimes be requested by young or childless couples who are certain that they do not want children. It is important to ask both partners to consider the following factors:

1. It should be looked upon as permanent and irreversible.

2. If their circumstances changed, e.g. financially or through the death of one of their children, might they want another child? It is probably unwise for a man to have a vasectomy if his youngest child is under two and the family of the size desired and no bigger.

3. If the wife died would the husband be likely to want children from another marriage?

4. How stable is their marriage? Does it seem likely that they might part and remarry?

5. Are there any sexual problems? If so, a vasectomy will make no difference except in so far as the need for contraception is concerned.

6. If the woman is on the pill, what are her periods like when she stops it? If they are very heavy and she is likely to want to go back on the pill or have a hysterectomy, the vasectomy would be unnecessary. It may be worth her while stopping the pill for three months to see what happens to her periods, using another method of contraception meanwhile.

7. Does either partner have any fear about the operation and its effects, however illogical? If either of them feel that it will in some way affect his manliness or sexual performance then it may be better for him not to have it done.

8. Contraception should be continued after the operation until the semen is found to be free of spermatazoa.

The vast majority of couples are well satisfied with the operation.

Difficulties sometimes arise in fat men or in those who have had previous surgery in the groin or scrotum. Sexual problems have been reported in those who also had them before the operation. Spermatazoa may persist in the seminal fluid for some months after the operation but eventually disappear except in those few who are eventually found to have a double vas or in whom the operation was inefficiently performed.

Women. Bilateral tubal ligation is a relatively safe and simple operation to perform but a general anaesthetic is required, and even with the fashionable laparoscopic method, a high degree of skill is needed. Even in the short term, it is not a procedure to be undertaken as lightly as vasectomy. In the long term, there is evidence that women who have had the operation are more likely than others to have menstrual problems later and even to need hysterectomy.

It is difficult to know whether these problems arise as a direct result of the operation or whether women who are sterilised are for other reasons more likely to have later menstrual difficulties. In any case the pros and cons should be discussed carefully and at length before the operation is recommended.

Abortion

The Abortion Act of 1967 allows termination of pregnancy up to 28 weeks provided one or more of certain criteria are fulfilled. These are that:

1. The continuance of the pregnancy would involve risk to the life of the pregnant woman greater than if the pregnancy were terminated.
2. The continuance of the pregnancy would involve risk of injury to the physical or mental health of the pregnant woman greater than if the pregnancy were terminated.
3. The continuance of the pregnancy would involve risk of injury to the physical or mental health of the existing child(ren) of the family of the pregnant woman greater than if the pregnancy were terminated.
4. There is substantial risk that if the child were born it would suffer from such physical or mental abnormalities as to be seriously handicapped.

In every case a form, HSA 1, has to be signed by two doctors, one of whom must be the operating practitioner, certifying that the criteria are fulfilled.

For most doctors, the act is completely unworkable. It is not possible to state that the criteria are satisfied without using personal, unscientific interpretations of their meaning unrelated to medical knowledge or experience. The only one remotely related to medical fact is that referring to the relative risks of allowing the pregnancy to continue or of terminating it. In fact, for most women, termination at an early stage involves less risk than a full-length pregnancy and confinement so that this is not a helpful condition as the wording stands.

Doctors are not in a position to pass judgement on the quality of life for families, other than their own, or to forecast what effect another child might have in any particular situation. Nothing in their training makes them fitted for this. Perhaps nothing could. In the circumstances all a doctor can do is to help the woman decide what she feels is best for her and her family. He may be able to shield her from pressure from parents or other relatives or refer her to a social worker or other helpful person in the area.

In effect, this is abortion on demand, that is, at the discretion of the patient. The only alternative is to have abortion at the discretion of two doctors. It is difficult to see how any two doctors could ever decide on the patient's behalf whether it is desirable for her to have a baby or not. The best they can do is support her in her decision.

As in all other fields the doctor has a duty to be well informed about the methods of termination currently in use, the risks, long-term effects, availability of the service and its cost, if any. If he feels unable to help the patient, he should refer her to a colleague who will. He should not try to impose his own opinions or moral views on the patient. They apply to him alone and are irrelevant to her. In some areas there is a social worker with a special interest in the problems of women with unplanned pregnancies who will see the patient and help her to arrive at a decision.

Conclusion

To summarise, the oral contraceptive is the method of choice for a healthy young woman, especially if she has heavy or painful periods; vasectomy is the method of choice for a couple with a stable marriage whose family is complete and who can both accept it; and the cap or condom with spermicide is useful post-partum, during lactation, pre-operatively, for casual sex and for couples who are separated for long periods. The IUCD and sterilisation of the woman may be useful in situations where none of the other methods can be used. Termination must always be the last resort and an admission of failure.

6 PREGNANCY, BIRTH AND POST-NATAL CARE

Antenatal Care

In the past, antenatal care has been a purely practical process aimed at preventing the physical complications of pregnancy and childbirth. It is now clear that it is impossible to achieve even this without attention to the emotional health of the woman, and that there are also purely emotional aspects of pregnancy which are at least as important to the future health of both mother and child as the physical ones.

Antenatal care is preparation for childbirth in its fullest sense. It concerns the present and future health and well being of both mother and child. It may involve the most advanced medical technology but this is wasted if attention to other less apparently exciting aspects of the work are left undone. It is no use enabling a woman to have a baby by reconstructing diseased fallopian tubes or carrying out intra-uterine transfusions if she then batters it because her emotional health has been neglected.

This is work which involves the whole primary health care team. It cannot easily be well done by any one individual or by a hospital out-patient department alone. At its best it is shared between the hospital and the primary health care team. The main aims are:

1. The physical and mental health of the mother during and after the pregnancy and confinement.

2. The normal development, growth and full-term delivery of a healthy baby.

3. The early establishment of a close and confident relationship between the child and both parents.

Early Stages – The First Trimester

Many women come to the surgery either from excitement or panic when their period is only a few days late. There is no way of confirming pregnancy at this stage but a pregnancy test can be arranged to be carried out at the appropriate time. The standard test is now a haemagglutination test. It becomes positive about four weeks after conception which in a woman with a 28-day cycle is likely to be six weeks after the first day of her last menstrual period. She should be warned that if the result is negative and she still has not had a period, the test should be repeated two weeks later. At this very early stage, even before it is

Pregnancy, Birth and Post-natal Care 71

certain she is pregnant, it is worthwhile to check with her that she does not smoke — if she does she must stop immediately — and is taking no medicines which are not absolutely essential. She should be advised not to have X-rays and to tell any doctor she sees for any other reason that she may be pregnant.

If she has not had rubella vaccine in the past or a previous positive result from a test for rubella antibodies, blood should be taken at this stage for this to be done. If she contracts rubella during the first 16 weeks and it is confirmed by rising titres of antibodies in successive samples, then the risks of foetal abnormality should be discussed and termination of pregnancy offered. If rubella occurs before eight weeks the risk of the foetus being abnormal is about 60 per cent. Once a positive pregnancy test is received the process of antenatal care may begin provided that the woman is not seeking termination.

At the first as at all succeeding visits, the work may be shared between the doctor, midwife, nurse and receptionist in whatever arrangement they find works best. Where the care is shared with a hospital, the initial examination and blood tests are often carried out there with a further visit at about 34 weeks.

It is helpful to have a separate page in the medical records for antenatal care. It is not sufficient to record observations only on a card carried by the woman herself. These are often lost or left at home and cannot include warning notes which the doctor may need to make to remind himself to watch for certain complications which may be too unlikely to worry the patient with. As well as basic identification, the antenatal sheet should contain the following information.

Family History. Especially of twins, diabetes, hypertension, epilepsy, spina bifida, congenital dislocation of the hip.

Personal History. Smoking habits, occupation, marital status. Accommodation — is it adequate, secure, permanent, overcrowded? Who will help at home when the baby is born?

Medical History. Illnesses, operations, accidents. Recent and present medication. Illness since conception.

Menstrual History. Date of last menstrual period and cycle length during last year. Has she recently stopped the oral contraceptive pill?

Obstetric History. Details of previous pregnancies and confinements including termination of pregnancy and miscarriages.

Emotional State. Was the pregnancy planned?
Is she pleased to be pregnant?
How much does she know about childbirth?
Is she afraid of the confinement?
How does she see herself as a mother?
Does she have doubts about her competence to care for or ability to love the child?
Is she looking forward to breast feeding?
How does she think her husband feels?
Will he come with her for some of her visits?
Will he be present when the baby is born?
Will they both attend classes for expectant parents?

This should be a leisurely interview so that the woman has plenty of time to express any fears or anxieties she may have and ask questions. At the end she should be told that there will be many other opportunities during the pregnancy to ask questions and discuss worries and that she should feel free to bring up any subject she likes at any of her antenatal visits.

The physical examination should include weight and height; examination of teeth, heart, breasts, legs, blood pressure; vaginal examination. Urine should be tested for sugar and albumen and an MSU sent to assess any bacteriuria. Blood should be taken for haemoglobin, ABO group, rhesus factor, rubella antibodies and serum test for syphilis, also for electrophoresis for abnormal haemoglobins in coloured women. Forms FP 24 and FW 8 should be completed. Arrangements for the confinement should be discussed with the patient even if there is not any real choice. It is a great help for a woman who already has a young child to stay in hospital for as short a time as possible and many units now have arrangements for 24-hour bookings.

Amniocentesis to exclude Down's Syndrome should be offered to any pregnant woman over the age of forty, but if she rejects termination of pregnancy on principle and therefore declines the test, no pressure should be brought to bear on her to agree. If the woman has had a previous baby or a close relative with spina bifida she should be offered alpha foetoprotein tests.

Unless there are obvious indications to the contrary, it should be made clear to the patient that the doctor assumes she will stop smoking, be healthy throughout the pregnancy, that the confinement will be normal, that her husband will be present and that she will breast feed. It should be obvious to her that plenty of help will be available at all stages.

It is usual to provide her with a prescription for iron and folic acid tablets at this visit but they are not essential and she may prefer not to start them until later if she is vomiting.

Vomiting in pregnancy can be the source of much misery. It is clear that it has emotional connections but it occurs in women who very much want the pregnancy and who do not seem fearful or anxious. It usually stops if the woman goes away from home to stay with a relative or is admitted to hospital. The well-established anti-emetics seem to be safe and may help but they have side-effects of drowsiness and dry mouth which are intolerable for some women. It is important to take repeated MSUs if the vomiting continues as it is often associated with urinary infection. It usually settles down by about 12-16 weeks but sometimes continues throughout the pregnancy. It is most important that a woman with this problem should be treated with sympathy and understanding and not as a neurotic idiot. The vomiting may make her feel very miserable and as though she has failed in not being healthily pregnant. This can be the start of loss of confidence which the primary health care team must take pains to counter.

The Second Trimester

From about 10-30 weeks it is usual to arrange antenatal visits to the surgery at monthly intervals. At each of these the weight and blood pressure are measured, the urine tested for albumen and sugar and the abdomen is examined. A note is made of the foetal movements and foetal heart once it can be heard. An ultrasound scan may be done to check the size of the foetus or exclude twins. It is also useful in showing the position of the placenta and in confirming the growth of the foetus. In some areas it is done routinely. At each visit the woman must have an opportunity of asking questions and expressing anxieties. Most women, especially primigravidae, are afraid of the confinement itself. They are afraid that it will be unbearably painful, that something will go wrong or that they will acquit themselves badly. It is not helpful to tell any woman that she will experience no pain but it does no harm to tell her that labour is painless for some women and that the staff will ensure that it never becomes more than she can stand. The emphasis is better laid on the hard work and boredom of labour which are usually present and easier to face than pain which is very variable. Information in this respect will be different in those areas where epidurals are available for all women in labour.

If she is worried about her capacity to love and mother a new baby, she should be reassured that this is a common anxiety and will pass in time but a note should be made so that the health visitor may watch for early difficulties particularly carefully. While encouraging her to plan to breast feed, care must be taken not to make her feel guilty if she eventually decides not to or fails in the attempt. The only thing that matters to the baby is that the mother is calm, relaxed and happy. If breast feeding worries or upsets her, it will not do the baby any good.

Anxieties about whether or not the baby will be normal are usual and should not be lightly dismissed. No one should be drawn into rash statements like 'I promise you the baby is normal.' The woman has to accept that no one can know for certain until it is born, but she can be reassured that there is no reason to suppose there is anything wrong.

If it is her first pregnancy, it may be useful to get her to talk about her husband's attitude and to mention that husbands sometimes seem to lose interest in their wives during pregnancy. She should realise that he may feel jealous of the baby or neglected by her if she is too tied up with it. If she realises that these difficulties are not unusual, she is likely to cope with them more effectively and with greater confidence.

If she already has another child, the effects on him of the pregnancy and of the forthcoming birth should be discussed. If she can be helped to see how devastating it can be for a toddler suddenly to have to share his mother, then she may be more tolerant of the problems he gives her and be able to protect him against the worst aspects of the situation. A form, Mat. B1, should be completed after 26 weeks.

The Third Trimester

At 30 to 32 weeks a further haemoglobin is done and blood taken for antibodies in rhesus-negative women. From this time on the visits are more frequent — every one or two weeks depending on the individual case. The pattern is the same as before but at this stage the position of the foetus and, in primiparae, engagement of the head are important.

It is quite common for the blood pressure to rise during the last few weeks of pregnancy. Provided the rise in both systolic and diastolic levels is slight and not accompanied by albuminuria and provided that it settles with rest at home, then no further treatment is necessary although it should be checked frequently. If the diastolic pressure rises to over 90 having previously been less than 80, or the systolic to over 130 having previously been less than 120 and does not fall again with rest, or if the woman cannot rest at home, she should be admitted to hospital.

Pregnancy, Birth and Post-natal Care 75

If weight is static for several weeks, or it seems that foetal growth is slow, placental function may be assessed by serial estimations of urinary oestradiol.

The Work of the Health Visitor

Parentcraft classes are best arranged by the health visitor at local level. This enables parents to get to know her and each other and allows the group to be small. Large groups run by a district hospital are impersonal, inhibit discussion and are much less successful. The class can cover whatever the group of potential parents and the organiser want it to. Films of childbirth are available and there can be practical demonstrations of bathing babies and mixing feeds. Other people, such as midwives or doctors, may be asked to join in with the discussions. The idea should be to encourage parents to stand on their own feet, to have the knowledge and confidence to care for their child in their own way, to know where to turn for help and advice if they need it and to do so without hesitation or shame. An important aim of the group is to help couples formulate their own ideas and perhaps try them out on each other. There is no reason why the group should not continue to meet after the babies are born if it can be arranged.

The health visitor should visit every woman during pregnancy if she possibly can. This allows them to get to know each other, the health visitor can form some idea of the mother's vulnerable points and where she is most likely to need help, and the mother can ask any outstanding questions that are bothering her and have the security of knowing the person who will be there to help her when she comes home with her baby. This is an opportunity for the health visitor to check that arrangements for the care of other children or elderly people in the house are satisfactory. She can arrange a home help if one is needed. She can check with the woman that she has everything she will need for the baby and that, if there are other children, they are prepared for what is going to happen.

If the woman is very poor, the health visitor may be able to provide her with baby clothes or other essential items and link her up with a social worker if she seems unable to cope or needs financial or other help.

The Normal Discomfort of Pregnancy

In a healthy woman pregnancy is a normal and natural state and need not alter a woman's way of life. She can continue with all her usual activities, including sex. She does not need more rest than anyone else, unless she is expecting twins, and should eat a normal diet. She may find she gains weight more easily than usual and should weigh herself regularly to ensure that she gains nothing before twelve weeks and not more than 1 lb a week on average after that, making a maximum total of 2 stones, rather less if she is short. During the early weeks, the breasts enlarge and become fuller with visible veins on the surface, there may be nausea and vomiting and frequency of micturition. She should not have vaginal bleeding, abdominal pain, dysuria or persistent or severe headache at any time during the pregnancy and should be warned to report any of these symptoms to her doctor.

Most women experience a feeling of breathlessness or difficulty in filling the lungs at some time in pregnancy. This is due to normal physiological changes and should be ignored. It is never severe.

During the later weeks it is common for there to be pain and tenderness along the lower chostochondral junctions. This is associated with pressure from the enlarging uterus and the resulting change in shape of the lower rib cage. It can be relieved by lying down. Sometimes a woman experiences a dramatic fall in blood pressure when lying on her back during the third trimester. The condition simulates shock and it may appear as though she has had a haemorrhage but it is immediately corrected by a change of position. It seems to be due to a reduction in venous return to the heart presumably from pressure on the inferior vena cava. It is more likely to frighten the doctor, when it happens when he is examining a woman in this position, than the woman herself, who will avoid the position if she knows it makes her feel uncomfortable.

For most women, the worst aspects of pregnancy are its length and the ungainliness of the last trimester, but some feel vaguely unwell throughout. Nausea and fatigue are the commonest problems and are difficult to combat. Urinary infection and anaemia should be excluded but there is little else that can be offered except sympathy.

Parturition

There is evidence that a woman is more likely to have a normal delivery if the confinement is conducted at home than in hospital, a good example of how emotional factors affect a woman's health and normal functioning. It is also clear that, if problems do arise, it is better to be in hospital if a disaster is to be avoided. This gives rise to much agonising both amongst women themselves and within the professions.

Most confinements are now conducted in hospital and the primary health care team is not directly involved, but some still take place in GP units and in some the district midwife, who has seen the woman during her pregnancy, looks after her in hospital, takes her home after 24 hours and continues to care for her. This continuity is very useful. The midwife can get to know her patient well and recognises signs of strain, depression or anxiety at an early stage. The mother is more easily able to relax and be calm and breast feeding flourishes. This is more difficult in a hospital ward where frequent changes of staff and the hospital routine make for a restless atmosphere, nervewracking to some women. However good the staff, each is not long enough in contact with a woman to be able to establish a trusting relationship and if such a relationship does begin, the woman's confidence is shattered when she finds that 'her nurse', who she is beginning to depend on, is off duty.

The closer the links between the primary health care team and the hospital, the easier it is for the lying-in period to be a natural sequel to the pregnancy and not a grim nightmare, or miserable sojourn, in an alien land. The 24-hour admission has much to recommend it and it seems a pity it is not used often for primigravidae. If the woman has to stay in for 8-10 days, then it helps if the health visitor goes to see her while she is there. They can plan together what will happen when the mother and baby go home and the fear and anxiety surrounding the prospect of being on her own with the baby can be shared and reduced.

The later development of a close relationship between mother and child depends to a great extent on early contact. The sooner she can hold her baby, preferably to the breast, or at least with their skins touching, the better. This early close contact is of the deepest emotional significance. It sows the seeds of maternal feeling even in those women least well endowed with this quality. Particular problems arise for women and babies deprived of this experience. A baby who remains in hospital after his mother is discharged is at risk of a permanently damaged relationship with her and even of being battered. The primary health care team should realise the existence of this risk factor in a family and do all they can to see that the problems are kept to a minimum. Help with transport may enable the woman to visit the baby frequently and even to continue to breast feed. Frequent visits from the health visitor during the early years and discussion of the mother's feelings may help to prevent the worst results of an early separation.

The foetus *in utero* is subjected to stress at an early stage. The most obvious factors are physical ones which cause disturbance of growth or development. These include virus infections, drugs, irradiation, smoking and alcohol. It is difficult to establish the effect of psychological stress on the foetus. It is said that the mother's state of mind during pregnancy influences how her baby will behave when he is first born. If she is anxious and tense during the pregnancy the baby cries a lot. He seems insecure and unsettled. He tends to suffer from colic, although whether this causes the crying or results from it is difficult to determine. It is certainly true that some babies are like this, while others are placid and contented from the beginning. The difficulty of proving a connection between maternal and foetal peace of mind arises from the fact that the mother's emotional state during pregnancy is likely to persist after her confinement. Then there is no doubt that it affects the baby.

The stressful effect on the baby of the process of birth is apparent. Whether it can be significantly reduced by dimmed lights, absolute quiet and super-gentle handling is doubtful. There is no evidence that the stress of birth is harmful to the baby born to a happy, relaxed mother. In fact it may be that this is the first hurdle which, if successfully handled, will enable the child to advance.

Post-natal Care

The first few weeks at home, after the birth of the baby, are particularly important. This is the time when the relationship between mother and child is established. The quality of their life together is influenced more by what happens now than at any other time apart from the initial contact. The mother is likely to be a victim of all sorts of conflicting emotions — love for the child, fear of hurting him or being unable to care for him, guilt that her love for him is not pure and unalloyed but diluted by resentment that he causes her so much anxiety and fatigue and has changed her life in so many ways. All these feelings are normal, but if they overwhelm her they affect the way she cares for the baby, and his awareness of her anxiety affects his own well being.

During early infancy the child becomes fractious with heat, cold, hunger, thirst, pain and discomfort. His reactions to these stimuli will be muted if he is happy and secure, exaggerated if he is tense and anxious. His state of mind reflects that of his mother. If she is anxious, tense or depressed, the child is restless and miserable. He cries a lot, especially at night. He appears to be in pain, drawing his legs up and screaming. He may overfeed and vomit. He fails to gain weight at a steady rate. He is excessively upset by minor difficulties and becomes progressively less able to deal with stress as he meets it. The more miserable the baby becomes the more the mother's anxiety grows, mixed with feelings of guilt from the realisation that she is in some way responsible for the baby's distress. She may resent the child and the unhappiness he is causing her. If she is breast feeding, she feels that her milk is not good enough and is not satisfying him. The mother's confused mixture of emotions involving fear, anger, love and guilt combined with physical fatigue causes great unhappiness for the whole family. Many women break down. Some batter their babies. It makes a poor start for the relationship between mother and child. If there is another child in the family it can be a time of great stress for him. Marital relationships suffer.

Helping families in this situation requires skill and experience. On the one hand the woman has to be enabled to understand the situation and to develop insight into her own contribution to the problem. On the other hand she needs reassurance about her ability to be a satisfactory mother and help in rebuilding her shattered self-confidence. She needs to understand what she is doing wrong in order to alter her own behaviour but must not be made to feel even more guilty. This is work at which health visitors usually excel. The aura of calm confidence which the good health visitor brings with her, the way in which she appears to have unlimited time for the problem in hand, however hardpressed she may be, her sympathetic attitude and sound practical advice are all enormously helpful.

Doctors, unfortunately, often make these situations worse. They are likely to be involved when the baby's crying and the mother's anxiety lead to the fear that the child has some physical illness. The situation may reach crisis point at night or weekend and be presented to the doctor as an acute emergency. He may already know that things are not going very well with this family and feels sure before he gets there that he is not going to find anything seriously wrong with the child. He saw the mother with the baby in the surgery last week and it was 'just a feeding problem'. He is brusque, irritated, impatient – in a hurry. He tells the parents there is nothing wrong and rushes off. This has a disastrous effect. The parents are made to feel foolish at having called him unnecessarily. Resentment against the child is increased. If there is nothing wrong, the child should not cry, yet he continues to cry. They can think of nothing else they can do. The doctor was their last hope and he has failed them.

Clearly the doctor cannot take the place of the health visitor and he should not try to. However, he can learn a lot from her technique and by doing so may well save himself time and trouble and the patient much distress. To begin with, when he sees the mother and child in the surgery at an early stage, he should be able to recognise the warning signs and take notice of them. The mother comes because the child cries. The doctor conscientiously looks for physical disease; he examines the ears, nose, throat, abdomen, hernial orifices. He finds nothing wrong. If this is all he does, he is storing up trouble for himself and the family. What else he does on this occasion may decide whether or not he gets that night call next week. This is his opportunity to ask in detail what the pattern of life is like for this mother and child. How much sleep does she get? Does she go out at all? What time does her husband come home? Where does her mother live? He may then comment on what a great strain it must be on her, being cooped up all day with a screaming baby, having had little sleep. He may think there is nothing he can do, but she will be immensely reassured that he appears to understand what it must be like for her, tells her that the baby is alright and will come to no harm through crying, that she is doing all she can for him. He should tell her that a lot of babies are like this and offer her some simple practical advice to take her through the next two or three days. He might suggest that she visit her sister, ask her mother to have the baby for a couple of hours, make some minor change in the feeding arrangements. He must promise to discuss the matter with the health visitor and ask her to call. He might warn the woman that she is likely to continue to have difficulties with the baby from time to time but they will get less. He should advise her to telephone him if she is worried, so that she does not wait for panic to develop before she calls him in the middle of the night. If he succeeds in reassuring her, she will become calmer and more confident and this will be communicated to the baby who will also relax.

This may sound time-consuming but it is surprising how much can be squeezed into a five or ten minute consultation. Appearing to be unhurried is not the same thing as spending a lot of time on a problem. To be of any use to the patient, the doctor must discard his traditional aura of busyness. He must be at pains to avoid implying that she should not have come to him with such a trivial problem, although it does no harm to suggest that the health visitor might be more help to her. Children seen years later, with behaviour problems and delinquency, frequently have a history of early difficulties with feeding and sleeping which were never satisfactorily resolved. The future of the child, and his ability to mature and handle stressful situations as he grows older, depends upon the satisfactory handling of early difficulties and the development of sound family relationships. The help he and his parents receive at this stage may be of critical importance.

The ability of all the members of the primary health care team to work together is especially useful during the puerperium. The woman's self-confidence is at its lowest ebb and yet she wants and needs help and advice which if given tactlessly, will diminish it still further. It is essential for the whole team to accept that the woman is likely to be emotionally frail and behave in an immature and sometimes silly way, asking questions to which she must already know the answers and needing endless support.

The receptionist can make or mar the whole relationship. If she shows surprise or incredulity that the woman wants the doctor to see her baby yet again (the third time in a week), the woman's self-confidence and equanimity may be destroyed. Her judgement must be respected as the best she can manage at the time. She can be tactfully channelled towards the health visitor, if this seems appropriate, but must never be scorned or belittled.

The post-natal examination is carried out by a doctor and traditionally includes a vaginal examination, to check that involution is complete, and nothing else. This is illogical as it is unlikely to yield any useful information and there are other important matters which are often omitted. Even if the uterus is not completely involuted by six weeks after the confinement, it is not usual to take any action, unless there is also abnormal bleeding or pain suggesting the presence of retained products or infection. The following practical procedures should be included at the post-natal visit: weight, blood pressure, mid-stream urine, examination of breasts, vaginal examination and cervical smear.

Contraception should be discussed and appropriate arrangements made. Most couples use a sheath during the first few post-partum weeks. A cap cannot be satisfactorily fitted until involution is complete and it seems preferable to allow the menstrual cycle to have returned before starting an oral contraceptive and to avoid it in women who are lactating. If a woman who is breast feeding is anxious to take the pill, she should be advised to wait until lactation is well established, and for most that means about ten weeks. A progestogen-only pill is a possible alternative.

Apart from arranging contraception, the most valuable part of the post-natal visit is the discussion about how the woman feels and how the baby is settling down and fitting in to the family. If she is simply asked if she has any problems she will probably say 'no', but if she is asked how often the baby wakes at night, whether she is tired, irritable or tearful and other specific questions, then a more complete picture will appear. Most women know enough to expect the post-natal blues during the first few days after the baby is born but few expect the depression to be as severe or as persistent as it often is, nor do they expect it to arise for the first time several weeks after the confinement.

Women are almost universally ashamed of post-natal depression. They cannot accept it as an illness beyond their control and feel guilty that they cannot be happy and grateful for a normal baby, loving husband, family and friends. This makes them hesitate to mention their depression even if it is quite severe. However, a woman will usually admit it if asked specifically and much useful work can be done by reassuring her that it is a common reaction and will pass if she is patient and not too self-critical.

If the depression is at all marked then it is important for a member of the primary health care team to maintain contact with the woman. The doctor may arrange for the health visitor to call on her the next day and perhaps ask her to telephone him at an agreed time a few days later. She may deteriorate rapidly and cannot be trusted to return if she does. Close co-operation between the general practitioner, health visitor and community psychiatric nurse is very useful in this situation.

In the absence of depression, the post-natal visit is a good time to talk about babies and their development. Few parents talk to their children enough or play with them at an early age. Many are embarrassed to do so, feeling that the child cannot possibly understand. If a more natural relationship between mother and child can be promoted, then they are likely to develop a close and loving bond at an early stage.

It is during the early months that the foundations of emotional development are laid. By fostering the sound relationship between mother and child, the members of the primary health care team can be instrumental in preventing emotional handicap and disability.

7 MARRIAGE

When it works well, the rather formal, long-term pairing of men and women in marriage is outstandingly successful. It has major benefits for the adults themselves, for society and especially for children. It is one of the most important factors influencing the health quotient. The frequency with which it fails shows that there are serious difficulties for many people in making marriage work.

Marriage as a Factor in Health

This is an important subject for the primary health care team. Many of the stresses which can weaken disease resistance and threaten health are most successfully overcome within the protective environment of a happy marriage. The vulnerability of both partners to setbacks at work, financial problems, emotional upsets and disease is reduced. Even a woman with an inauspicious upbringing can overcome her disadvantages if she and her husband build a stable marriage. Children in a home based on a successful marriage are not only healthier but are more likely to carry their capacity for health into adult life. Their ability to form successful, mature, adult relationships will be high and their own marriages will be more likely to succeed.

The amount of ill health directly related to marital misery is inestimable. A large number of people attend doctors' surgeries every day seeking relief from emotional symptoms, depression or anxiety related to it. Others need help as a result of physical violence. Many of those affected do not see a doctor or if they do, keep the cause of their trouble to themselves. As well as these there are many who find minor illness or other problems insupportable because of the debilitating affect of their overall unhappiness, who find themselves unable to cope with normal stresses because their defences are weakened. There are yet others who develop purely neurotic symptoms related to the stress of domestic disharmony. A high proportion of attempted suicides have the same basis. Alcoholism results from marital problems as well as causing them. Resistance to disease and accidents of all sorts is higher in people under stress. Marital disharmony is the most devastating kind of stress and one which affects all the members of the family.

Marriage Counselling by the Health Team

Whether the primary health care team consists of a single-handed doctor and one district nurse or a full team including community psychiatric nurse, social worker and marriage guidance counsellor, its members will find themselves doing a certain amount of marriage counselling whether they want to or not. Even if he is thoroughly fed up with her and feels unable to help, the doctor must hear out the distraught woman whose marriage is in tatters and make comforting noises to go with his prescription for valium. If he denies that marital problems are part of his job, he still has to see and treat, if he can, the illness and disability which result from them. The work they do is likely to be more interesting and more effective if the members of the team undertake it with enthusiasm, a clear idea of what they hope to achieve and of their own limitations. Marriage counselling is complex and skilled and requires training, as well as natural ability, if it is to be done well. Those teams who have a marriage guidance counsellor as one of their members are at a great advantage. Not only can she undertake much of the work herself but other members benefit from her expertise and experience. It is not possible for all the marriage counselling in a practice to be undertaken by a skilled and trained marriage guidance counsellor. Some of the couples needing help will not see her and will accept help only from the health visitor or doctor. Some of the most useful work in stimulating a couple to seek help has to be done by whoever is in contact with them at the time and recognises their need. Counselling is most likely to be helpful if it is sought by a couple at an early stage in their difficulties but at this point they may be unaware that it might help them. It is therefore useful for all members of the team to take an interest in and develop some skill in recognising marital problems.

The Basis of a Successful Marriage

It may be useful first to examine some aspects of marriage. Couples entering into it need to be as mature as possible and those marrying very young are less likely to make a success of it. They should both want to marry solely because they love each other and want to spend the rest of their lives together, and not because they are under pressure from their parents, want to get away from home, or because the girl is pregnant. It is a great help if they have somewhere to live or at least the prospect of a home and are not going to have to live with parents for a prolonged period. Shortage of accommodation for single people and for newlywed couples is a serious problem.

The most important factors influencing the future success of the marriage are the personalities of the couple, their attitude to themselves and each other and their expectations of marriage. No couple can live permanently in a romantic haze of domestic bliss. It would probably be very dull. The happiest will have blazing rows from time to time and none will succeed without hard work and determination. There are recurring areas of conflict in every relationship and the couple must be prepared to work to understand and overcome the difficulties which inevitably arise. The advantage of marriage is that it provides a relatively secure environment within which quarrels can occur without threatening the stability of the whole.

Anything that can be said about marriage also applies to long-term relationships not based on marriage and to homosexual relationships. To succeed, any of these must be based on mutual love and respect and flexible expectations of what the relationship can provide. Each partner has to have a belief in the equal value of both regardless of the role each plays at home and in the community. It is no help for them both to agree that the wife and her work are less important than the husband and his. As much harm is done to the relationship by her undervaluing herself as by him having an inflated view of himself. The woman has to have self-respect and status in her own eyes if she is to contribute equally to the partnership. If she underrates herself, she will see her work, interests and friends as less important than her husband's and will neglect them. She will then be entirely dependent on him for all her intellectual, social and emotional needs which he cannot possibly satisfy. She will look upon her own sexual satisfaction as less important than his and their sex life will be unsatisfying to both. Whatever the man's initial attitude it will be difficult for him to persist in looking upon his wife as his equal if she does not do so herself. He will begin to take her for granted, lose respect for her and treat her like a servant. Marriage cannot succeed in this situation. The commitment to equal value may be difficult to achieve because society as a whole sets a lower value on women and their work than on men, and the partners bring with them to the marriage the effects of a socialisation process based on this tradition. This is a very subtle force. Many couples who claim to see each other as equals belie this in their behaviour. The woman's need for sexual satisfaction is given a low priority, if recognised at all. Her interests and hobbies are tolerated but disparaged, his are important. If she is a full-time housewife, the family income is seen as his salary out of which she receives a housekeeping allowance. However generous this is, she has no money in her own right. He keeps up with his friends, plays football or golf, while she cares for the children during evenings and weekends. The family hobbies reflect his interests. He belongs to an all-male club with specially arranged activities for wives. If both work full time, the household chores are her responsibility with which he 'helps', often with startling ineptitude. Her income is looked on as pocket-money however important it is in fact.

Couples who cannot escape the influence of their upbringing and put the equality-of-value principle into full effect, can achieve a great deal if they agree that equal value is what they believe should operate and what they will work towards. Then, when they find themselves slipping away from it, they can correct the tendency. If this commitment is made, then the other requirement, flexibility of expectation, is much easier to achieve. On a purely practical level, a man who truly respects the importance of his wife's interests finds no difficulty in agreeing to care for the children and prepare their tea when she is playing in a hockey match on a Saturday afternoon. A self-respecting woman will continue to meet her friends and keep up her own interests so that she will not mind when her husband comes home from work tired and uncommunicative, wishing only to relax in a chair for a while. She may well feel the same. For partners to be of equal value within a marriage does not mean that they have also to be of equal dominance. It is common for one or other to be the dominant partner and need not lead to insuperable problems as long as the situation is understood and accepted.

Most marriages in this country are founded on the basis of romantic love, that is a combination of sexual attraction and emotional interdependence. In marriages that succeed and last this romantic love grows and develops into something much more solid and deep-rooted than it is at the beginning. The partners become complementary and necessary to each other so that even if there are fluctuations in the intensity of their romantic attachment, the marriage itself is never threatened. The relationship between them changes and develops, steadily growing stronger. Static marriages where the relationship does not change or gets stuck at a particular point are much more vulnerable and likely to break down or die of boredom. The degree of interdependence is important. To love someone is to be dependent on that person to some extent, but if one partner is too dependent on the other, or if there is a great difference between the amount of dependence each has on the other, then complex difficulties can arise.

No two people can ever provide entirely for each other's needs at all levels throughout their lives. It is a mistake to try and only leads to disappointment and feelings of guilt and resentment when the inevitable result is failure. People change as they grow older and things which at one time seem unimportant become necessary later on. Couples become dissatisfied if they depend on each other for everything. A commitment to the equal-value principle allows each to seek social and intellectual stimulation outside the marriage as well as within it. This principle is much more difficult to apply to sexual needs. Human sexual activity is inseparably linked with love and within marriage becomes an expression of that love. Unless there are serious sexual problems within the marriage, sex without love with an outsider is not particularly tempting and therefore all extra-marital sex implies emotional involvement and is a threat to the marriage. For most couples sexual fidelity is necessary to marital harmony.

Although most couples now set up home on their own, forming a nuclear family separate from their extended family, the relationships they have with their parents and siblings and even more distant members of the family may be of the utmost importance in their marriage. A young adult who has not grown out of the childish dependence on his parents, perhaps because one of them has been domineering or smothered him so that he could not mature normally, will find it very difficult to form a marital relationship. The influence of parents on the interactions of a couple within marriage can be complex and destructive.

There are several different aspects to the work of the primary health care team in this field. There may be opportunities to influence attitudes of groups of children in school as well as individual adolescents at the surgery to themselves, each other and marriage. Early marriage might be discouraged. There is no way of knowing how far this is possible but at least the attempt should be made.

Individuals may seek premarital counselling but it is sometimes also well received by those coming to the surgery for another reason such as contraceptive advice or to request termination of pregnancy. If they can be encouraged to talk about their own feelings and views about marriage they can sometimes be enabled to resist pressures to marry too young or against their own judgement. If they have problems at home or need accommodation, the social worker may be able to help so that marriage is not the only way out of what they see as an intolerable situation.

Discussion groups for engaged couples are already run in some areas by marriage guidance counsellors or the church. This could be extended with the primary health care team as a base where this is convenient. Such groups could continue to meet after marriage and identify problem areas as they arise. Marriage could be included in the subjects to be discussed by groups of school leavers or youth club members. The local vicar and members of the primary health care team would be valuable assets in such groups provided they avoided the temptation to lecture.

Helping a Marriage in Difficulty

The best time to help a marriage in difficulties is before they have become serious. To do this it must be widely known in the community that this help is available. A marriage guidance counsellor working as part of the team may be in a better position to attract couples to seek help at this early stage. Too often marriage guidance is viewed as a last resort and not sought until the breakdown has already happened. The members of the team may be able to identify those couples likely to have problems well in advance and make sure that they are offered help as soon as they feel able to accept it.

Among those particularly at risk are those who marry young, those who have several children under school age, and those where the woman is socially isolated. Where either partner has been to a single-sex boarding school and where they come from widely different cultural backgrounds, the marriage is more likely to break down and also if the partners are separated for long periods. Particular problems arise when one partner has an emotionally exhausting job. Doctors and social workers come into this group. They may not have sufficient emotional resources to keep both the job and the marriage going and often lack the insight to realise that the marriage is under strain or even breaking up.

As with many other aspects of health care, this work may be undertaken by different members of the team depending upon their interests, availability, training and the choice of the patient. Whoever is doing it and at whatever stage of marital difficulty the problem is presented, it is a great advantage if both partners can be seen together. This is hardly ever possible at first but where marriage guidance counsellors are members of the teams couples may be more willing to come together. The aim of marital counselling is to enable the couple to identify the basis of their problems and to reach solutions for themselves. It is no help for them to hear what the counsellor thinks they should do. However sensible the advice, it can only be given from the counsellor's point of view and will always contain elements of 'what I would do if I were you' which are totally irrelevant. The counsellor's role should be to open up for them areas in their relationship of which they are unaware or which they have not previously discussed and to encourage each to face those things about himself which make life difficult for the other.

Once these things have been admitted and discussed they may be easier to tolerate even if they cannot be changed.

Flexibility depends on emotional maturity and a stable personality. These can only develop in someone who has had a secure and happy childhood with stable relationships from an early age. Many adults lack this background and the counsellor must accept that their ability to change their attitudes and behaviour may be limited. It may be clear to everyone including the people themselves what would be best for them to do but if this involves making changes which for them are impossible, then this is not one of the options open to them. To attempt it will lead to failure.

The difficulties many men have in discussing serious or emotional subjects often cause problems. Sometimes it is because the subject, for instance a sexual problem or heavy drinking, implies criticism of the man and he finds it threatening, but more often it is because his ability to communicate verbally is poor. It is common for a woman in describing her difficulties to complain that her husband 'will not discuss it'. If he can be enabled to admit that this is a problem he has, understand that his wife finds it difficult to live with, and resolve to work on it, then she may be able to be more tolerant of it.

Some of the most shattering crises occur in marriages of perhaps fifteen or twenty years' standing which one partner may describe as having been blissfully happy. 'We had no problems, we had always been happy and then he suddenly left, says he has fallen in love with someone else.' It is usually the man who leaves, but women do so as well and more often would like to but stay because of the children.

It is clear that in some cases such a marriage has not been so satisfying to one partner as the other believes. It is possible for two people to live together for many years without ever getting to know and understand each other very well, for the initial excitement of romantic love to have died and not been replaced by any more lasting attachment. Marriage is then just a habit. The man may have been sexually bored and irritated by his wife for some time. He may not have been aware of it until he meets someone else who appears to offer an exciting alternative. His wife also may have been unaware of his discontent or suppressed her recognition of it. If the marriage really has a weak foundation, then it may be impossible to rebuild it but sometimes a crisis such as this brings home to both partners that there is a depth of feeling between them which they had failed to recognise but which could be used to build a marriage, different from the one they had before and much more exciting and interesting. This is where the skilled counsellor can be a great help.

Even with a solid basis of mutual love and respect, marriage can make people miserable if it is not nurtured and difficulties identified and sorted out as they arise. Sexual boredom is a common problem. Couples may be inhibited in their willingness to experiment at home but may be able to do so on holiday on their own: even a weekend in a tent can be refreshing. Anger and resentment often builds up over difficulties in communication. A woman may seem to be unreasonably angry when her husband forgets a trivial matter or is reluctant to carry out some minor maintenance job in the house, but if she sees this as a rejection of her and their home then her anger is easier to understand. The wife of a quiet man who withdraws into a world of his own is more likely to become depressed as a result of his behaviour than the one whose husband sometimes hits her. Silent violence can be devastating.

Couples with Children

Couples with children need to take some trouble to be alone together regularly. However happy family life, they need to be reminded of the pleasure of each other's company.

It is too easy for a full-time housewife to become a drudge and never leave the house except to go shopping. For most women housework is boring, unrewarding and repetitive and little children are poor company. While she should make every effort not to let this happen, an occasional frivolous outing with her husband can be a useful antidote and serve to remind him that she is more fun to be with and just as glamorous as the women he meets at work.

Throughout the time that a couple are bringing up children, their own relationship must be of supreme importance. It is easy for it to be neglected when family life is busy and tiring but the risks of such neglect cannot be overstated. The ability of the children to grow and develop the capacity for satisfactory adult relationships is related to the quality of their parents' marriage. Not only do they observe it and use it as a model for themselves but their own emotional development is dependent on it. If the parents' relationship is not mutually satisfying, they are more likely to become overdependent on the children and in turn make it difficult for them to grow up and establish their own independence. Marital problems can often be traced back to the difficulty one or other partner had in breaking free from the powerful influence of one or both parents. If the neglect of the marriage leads to breakdown, separation or divorce then the children are permanently damaged.

In addition to the effects on the children, the couple should remember that they will have longer together after the children have grown up than before and if the marriage is to survive until this time then it should not be neglected during the early years.

If a marriage has already broken down and the couple clearly lack the will or the resources to rebuild it, the counsellor can be useful in helping them to separate and divorce, if that is what they want, with the minimum of bitterness and damage to family relationships. There is bound to be a great deal of unhappiness on both sides. Each will blame the other and at the same time feel guilty at the failure of the marriage. Both will be worse off financially and one or both will have to leave the family home. This leads to anger and resentment. The effect on children is always disastrous. This does not mean that divorce should be avoided at all costs when there are children. It may be better than struggling on with the family misery which springs from constant marital disharmony. It is nevertheless impossible for parents to separate without having a serious disruptive effect on the lives of the children. This has to be faced and the damage kept to a minimum. Children need to know and be able to love and respect both parents even if those parents do not love and respect each other and do not live together. Their ability to grow up and make satisfactory relationships themselves depends on this. In the early stages of marital breakdown the worst aspects for the children are the anxiety and insecurity which results from wondering what is happening, the fear for the future and the feeling that they are in some way to blame for it all. Parents should be encouraged to tell the children as much as possible without involving them in the dispute. They should never be allowed to take sides and both parents should resist the temptation to use a child as a confidant and comforter. It may help the mother but it does inestimable damage to the child to be told that his father is wicked and cruel and makes her unhappy. The children should be assured that they are in no way to blame either by simply existing or by anything they have done.

It is a great help if the couple can look upon the breakdown of the marriage as the failure of a partnership: a joint venture, a joint failure, to share the blame and try to retain mutual respect and remember what they once felt for each other. The counsellor may be able to encourage this attitude and should avoid the temptation to criticise either partner or take sides in the dispute.

After the couple have separated, the main concern should still be for the children. They should continue to see both parents and if possible spend extended periods with whichever one they do not live with. Both parents need tremendous self-control if each is to foster the love and respect of the children for the other. They have to suppress their own anger and bitterness and be prepared to take a share of the blame they do not feel. In later years, the children will appreciate this and their ties with both their parents will be stronger.

There may be opportunities for counsellors to talk to children themselves and encourage them to express their feelings. It may help a child to hear the outsider express liking or admiration for both parents.

8 FAMILY LIFE

Thoughts of children occupy an important place in the life of every married couple from the start. Even if they decide very definitely that they do not want to have any, they will spend some time coming to this decision and justifying it to themselves, their family and friends. Some couples decide to postpone starting a family for a few years and during this time wonder if they are doing the right thing and whether they will conceive when they want to. Some are already pregnant when they marry or conceive immediately after. Others want to have children, seem unable to achieve a pregnancy and wonder whether and how to adopt. Whatever their situation, the subject is ever present and for some people it is a source of anxiety and stress which may lead them to seek advice. As in all other counselling situations, the role of the professional is to help the couple to sort out their own difficulties and find their own solutions but there are certain general principles which may be useful in helping them to do this.

The Decision to Have Children

As with marriage itself, a couple should have a baby deliberately only if they really want one and not because they think they should or to please their parents, prove that they can or because they think that it might improve their marriage. Every couple has a moral duty to provide a child with the best start in life that they can manage. It is irresponsible deliberately to conceive when a marriage is unstable or likely to break down. Having a baby imposes an added strain on a marriage and is therefore unlikely to bring together a couple who are drifting apart.

Marriages of very young couples are less likely to last and very young women are more likely to have premature babies, perinatal and neonatal deaths and to lose a baby in the first year of life than those in their twenties. They should therefore consider waiting until their twenties before starting a family.

There are some couples who really do not want children but who feel under pressure from family, friends or society in general to conform to the standard pattern. It is most unwise for them to do so and they should be given every encouragement to recognise and stand by their own feelings and do what is best for them. The woman's guilt at lacking the maternal feeling she thinks she should have can cause her great distress and lead her to decide to put it to the test and have a baby she really does not want.

Older couples may seek information about the risks of pregnancy and foetal abnormality. After about the age of twenty-five, the risks of a first pregnancy increase with age and by the age of thirty-five are high enough to be discouraging. The risks of foetal abnormality also increase with age and women over the age of forty should think very carefully before embarking on a pregnancy even if it is not their first.

Loving the Baby

Whether the pregnancy was planned or not, once the baby is born the parents have to try to love and accept him. Any preconceived ideas or expectations about his sex, looks, behaviour and later on his achievements are replaced by sheer joy at his existence. It is only by adopting this attitude and allowing themselves to love the child wholeheartedly for his own sake that the right environment for emotional growth and development can be provided. Social and family pressures and the effects of their own upbringing make it difficult for parents to treat their child naturally. They are plagued by fears for the future, fears that he may develop badly and that it will be their fault. This makes them self-conscious in the way they handle him. They fear that if they cuddle him when he cries, he will become spoilt, demanding, even delinquent. If they cuddle him close naked, then his future sexuality may be endangered. As he grows there is an excessive preoccupation with obedience, the idea being that a child who has been subjected to discipline at an early age will work harder at school, have greater success and not kick over the traces. There is no evidence for this. What facts there are suggest that a child's future success depends upon secure, loving, close relationships with his parents in infancy. This is what the members of the primary health care team should aim to foster.

The health visitor and doctor should play down the importance of their own role in giving advice and use every opportunity to encourage the parents to behave instinctively towards the baby. They will then feel free to have pleasure in frequent close physical contact with him, talk to him, play with him, feed him when he is hungry, warm him when he is cold, comfort him when he is sad. They will become more natural and self-confident. Breast feeding will continue until the mother gets fed up with it or the baby bites the nipple or spits it out and demands something else. Weaning will start by the baby having tastes of different foods from his mother's plate. He will sleep when he is tired, eat when he is hungry, cry when he is uncomfortable or lonely. The

Family Life

mother is attuned to the baby, his needs and his normal behaviour. If he is unusually quiet, she will recognise this as abnormal and will seek help, possibly avoiding a cot death due to infection.

The baby absorbs and reflects the love of his parents and his natural inclination at all times is to please them. He feels totally secure. When he wakes in the night, he watches the shadows, plays with the sides of his cot or his blankets. He may hum or babble. He will not cry out unless he is uncomfortable and will soon settle again if changed and tucked up. If he is unwell or in pain from teething he may need comforting for a while during the night and his parents may prefer to take him into their bed. When he is back to normal he will be happy to stay on his own again. Problems are few and easily overcome. Family life is happy and relaxed.

As he becomes mobile, he will be protected from danger: he is not left alone, windows have safety catches or bars, the fire is guarded, plugs covered. He discovers that his actions have results and he learns by these. If he hits himself with a toy, it hurts and he learns not to do it again. Later, if he throws his food about his mother removes it. If he climbs dangerously high on the furniture, she is cross. When she feels he is ready for toilet training, she will show him a potty, indicate what it is for and wait until he shows some interest in using it. If he does, she is pleased and he will want to do it again. If he does not seem ready, she will be happy to wait. She accepts him and respects him, has no sense of disappointment at his refusal to perform and makes no attempt to persuade him. Even at this early age, his decision is respected. He is only overruled in matters of safety or important things which affect the lives of other members of the family and opportunities for these are kept to a minimum. If an older child wants to paint, he does it out of reach of the toddler or when he is asleep, or out, or in another room. If the toddler refuses to have his coat on when the family are going out on a cold day, the mother does not have a battle with him but takes the coat with her to put on later when he is cold. It is easy and pleasant for him to do what his parents want and so he becomes naturally obedient.

These parents find the child wants to please them and avoid their displeasure. They do not demand obedience for its own sake and therefore have little use for the concept of naughtiness. The emphasis is on co-operation. The relationship between parents and child is rather like the adult sexual relationship. It is something they all do together as equal partners, finding out what pleases each and building on the foundation of love and joy which the mutual interaction brings them all.

Within the security of this relationship, they can all safely assume that each desires to please the other if he or she possibly can. Failure to do so will upset the one causing them displeasure as much as the others. If the child causes his mother to be angry, he will be as upset as she and she recognises this. Punishment, apart from the natural withholding of approval for dangerous or antisocial behaviour, is irrelevant and unnecessary.

In this family tensions are at a minimum. Motherhood is interesting, pleasurable and fulfilling. The whole family has a high health quotient.

There is no incentive for this child to break out and experiment with outrageous behaviour when later he is no longer constantly supervised. Throughout he has been doing what pleased him. He has no sense of repression, no urge to misbehave.

Tensions Between Parents and the Baby

Problems arise when parents are unable to identify and follow their instincts. They cannot accept and love the baby as he is because they are harrassed by their expectations of what he should be like. His sleeping habits, feeding and all aspects of his behaviour are expected to conform to an arbitrary pattern unrelated to his natural tendency. They lose the sensual pleasure of having him and the joy of his response to them and theirs to him because they are set about by fears. They are anxious if he cries at night, rejects certain foods or continues to demand a breast feed when he 'should' have given it up. They try to mould his behaviour, to make him conform to the accepted pattern and are disappointed when he does not. He, sensing their displeasure, feels insecure. He cries more and is restless at night. If his parents are firm with him, make him stay in his own bed and leave him to cry, he becomes distraught. The child's basic need, to have his cry for help answered, is being denied. If they take him into bed with them, they are starting a habit which may be difficult to break. Unlike the happy, secure child, he will be unwilling to return to his own bed later. His pain will not get better like the pain of teething. His pain will last all his life.

There is no naturalness in the mutual response between parents and child, no pure delight. The basis of the relationship is no longer the mutual exchange of love and pleasure. The baby does not know how to please his parents. He becomes irritable and perverse. The concept of naughtiness creeps into the family relationships. Just as the Victorian husband imposed sex on his wife, these parents impose obedience on their child. The relationship is something to be suffered now and escaped from later. Obedience is what the child does, when he has to, when he is being watched. There is no pleasure in being obedient, only pain in

Family Life

doing wrong. He therefore misbehaves whenever he feels he may get away with it or when, in his anger and frustration, he wants to anger his parents. As their positive demonstrations of love and approbation lessen, anger may be the strongest emotion directed at himself that he can elicit. In the absence of love it may be better than nothing. The mother is not attuned to this baby and if he is unusually quiet she thinks he is being 'good' at last.

There are a number of reasons why a child may refuse to use a potty, go to bed or eat food that he is expected to. The more pressure he is under, the more complex these reasons become. His behaviour is nearly always interpreted as naughtiness and punished. Punishment in this situation is not the natural result of certain behaviour, which he can modify, but an incomprehensible and unconnected external force adding to his misery. He then becomes more unwilling, even unable, to co-operate and the problems increase.

Tensions in the Family

The tensions in this family are enormous. The mother has all the drudgery of housework, the tedium of caring for a baby with little adult company and none of the rewards of maternity. She is deprived of the joy of a mutually fulfilling, loving relationship with the child. She feels angry with him because he is naughty, resentful at her deprivation and guilty about these feelings and about her obvious failure as a mother. She is frustrated and helpless, tired, anxious, depressed. The baby is immediately aware of how she feels and is miserable and demanding. He is hard to please. He may be deliberately naughty to gain her attention. If the tension rises enough, she may batter him.

Her husband escapes during the day, although he carries some of the family anxiety with him to work. When he returns, there is no joy to greet him, only tears and tiredness: an irritable baby and an exhausted wife. After a while he may work late or stop off for a drink on the way home to steel himself for the ordeal. This adds fuel to the inevitable row which follows. She has no time or energy to keep up with her friends or follow independent interests. She is overwhelmed by the difficulty of looking after the baby. All day is spent looking forward to her husband coming home in the evening. She looks to him not only for comfort, company and intellectual stimulation but also for an answer to her problems. When he arrives, all her pent-up frustration overflows into a quarrel. He and the baby have both let her down. There is no possibility of them all working together to their mutual advantage.

This child grows up as if he is among strangers. He lacks the secure knowledge of his parents' love. He never learns the pleasure of pleasing them. Their love seems to him conditional on his good behaviour and therefore not real or worth having. His ability to form mature relationships when he grows up is limited. He is an emotional cripple. The health quotient of the family is at its lowest.

Helping the Troubled Family

There are numerous occasions when members of the team are in contact with mothers and young children. They are seen by doctor and midwife during the puerperium, by the health visitor frequently during the first year and regularly until the child is five years old, by the doctor at the post-natal visit, well-baby and immunisation sessions, apart from any visits for problems or illness.

While some women are perfect natural mothers and need no help and others seem unable to respond to any, there are a large number who are able to benefit from contact with the right person at the right time. Some find it difficult to recognise their natural instincts, others lack the self-confidence to follow them, others are overwhelmed by pressures from parents or in-laws. Some are emotionally reserved or inhibited as a result of their own childhood experiences. It should be possible to help all these; to expand their horizons to some extent, to increase their options so that they are less severely limited in their choice of actions, to free them from some of the bonds that society and their upbringing has placed on them. However, professional advice can serve to make their problems worse. If a mother is told how to care for her baby, how he should behave, what she should be feeling, she will have yet another set of external standards to live up to, another set of expectations. She will have her confidence in her own ability to care for the child without help even further undermined. She will be confused by the different advice she receives from different people and made anxious because it all conflicts with her natural inclination. Her natural instincts are even more difficult to recognise let alone follow. Totally instinctive behaviour in a human mother is not possible because it is too heavily overlaid by generations of socialisation. A woman in a modern Western society cannot and would not want to deliver her own baby, eat the placenta, suckle and care for the child entirely without help. There are great benefits to be gained from civilisation but it must not be allowed to overwhelm the woman so that she and her baby fail to develop a proper relationship. Attempts should be made to retain and foster as much as possible of their natural instincts and behaviour.

When professional workers give instructions to a new mother they should be confined to technical matters, on which she may be expected to need information and which she is unlikely to know already. This will include how to mix artificial feeds, sterilise bottles, fold nappies. In all other matters the advice should be completely non-directional. The woman should be encouraged to do what she thinks is right and be supported in doing so. She may have difficulty in sorting out what she wants to do from the mass of advice she has heard and read. She may need to discuss her ideas in order to formulate them and it may help her to hear of the health visitor's experience or even relevant anecdotes, but she should never be told what to do. If she is given precise instructions as to how to handle her baby, she is unlikely to be able to carry them out and will feel anxious and frustrated. No set of instructions apply to every situation, every woman, every baby, and they cannot be tailor-made. The woman and the baby have to work out for themselves what methods suit them best. In any case, no two days are the same and flexibility is essential even within one family.

A well-baby clinic is a good opportunity for a mother to seek the help and support of a health visitor without waiting for a problem to arise. She should be encouraged to attend because she might like a chat and to show off her baby rather than because the health visitor thinks she is incompetent to care for the child on her own. Everything she is doing should be commended and the baby admired unreservedly even if the health visitor also adds some suggestions which she might like to try. By her own attitude towards the child, the health visitor may be able to break down some of the woman's inhibitions. She can show that there is nothing silly or undignified about talking to a baby, nothing reprehensible in enjoying the feel of its skin. These things are normal. The baby clinic offers a valuable opportunity for mothers and babies to meet each other. They may have met already at the antenatal clinic or elsewhere in the community. This is another chance to make friends, exchange notes and talk to someone other than child or husband.

If developmental examinations by a doctor are carried out, they should be to support the mother and appreciate the progress she and the baby are making rather than solely to look for something wrong with the baby. They should be an opportunity for her to discuss any difficulties or anxieties she has and plans for the future. If she is anxious about his weight, it may be useful to show her where it lies on a percentile chart. A sleeping problem may be difficult to influence but it may help the mother to tolerate it better if she can talk about it and be reassured that there is nothing wrong with the child, and that she will do no harm by taking him into bed with her sometimes if that is what she wants to do. It may be possible to enlighten her as to the link between a toddler's refusal to stay in his own bed and the arrival of the new baby. If she can see how desperate he may be feeling, she may be able to soften her attitude to his 'naughtiness' and find him more time during the day and at bedtime to demonstrate her love for him. When a doctor says 'Of course toddlers are into everything, I expect there are times when you find you haven't said a kind word to him all day', there is sometimes a flash of recognition in the mother, as she sees herself constantly grumbling at the mobile, active two-year-old, while she is never cross with the baby.

As with marital problems, the counsellor's role is partly to enable the couple, that is the mother and the child, to see aspects of themselves and their situation of which they had previously been unaware.

Sources of Stress

Toilet training and nocturnal enuresis are the source of much family stress. They should be viewed as things the mother and child work at together, in partnership, and not as something the mother imposes on the child. It should be assumed that the child wants to be dry and clean even if only (at first) to please his mother, and that he will do it as soon as he can. If a schoolchild waking to a wet bed can be met with 'don't worry darling, I'll put the sheets in the washing machine, while you have a wash down', the child at least feels she is on his side.

It is easier to absorb a new baby into a family if the previous one is over three and a half or four years old. By this time his position is secure, he will be toilet trained even if he is not dry at night and his eating and sleeping habits are stable and accepted. He will probably be attending a playgroup or nursery school. He will enjoy the new baby without feeling unduly threatened, and will be able to continue with the special relationship with his parents which has been already established. He will find it easy to be loving and tolerant towards the new baby. It is not impossible for a new baby to arrive without upsetting the family if the first child is much younger than this, but it is certainly more difficult and an added strain on the mother and toddler. No member of the primary health care team will ever want to try to tell a couple how they should space their children, but parents are often unaware of the problems a second baby may bring and are interested to hear the experience of the health visitor or other worker.

The Child's Development in the Early Years

The pattern of family life which follows the arrival of the first baby

Family Life 101

stems from the relationship founded during his early years. If they are based on mutual love and respect and the desire to please, then the child and his parents grow, develop and mature together without serious difficulty. Secure in his position in the family, he begins to develop emotional as well as physical independence. He accepts a new baby with a minimum of fuss. He is enthusiastic for new experiences and happy to go to school. He tackles new tasks with enthusiasm, knowing that his parents will take pleasure in his success, comfort him in failure. They want for him only what will make him happy and what he wants for himself. They are in no danger of developing unrealistic expectations of him. Their ambitions for him at school are that he should be happy, make successful relationships and make use of his natural talents so that he fulfils his potential. If they are fortunate, the school will have a similar outlook based on the principle of equal value,[1] respect for the individual and co-operation in work, but even if it has not, he is now secure and flexible enough to be able, with his parents' support, to understand and put up with different attitudes at school to those he is used to at home.

He is now able to understand and even benefit from observing, or being the object of, his parents' anger. It is reassuring to know that they, whom he respects and admires, are sometimes subject, as he is, to painful, passionate feelings, which are difficult to control and which they later regret, but which do not alter their love for him. They should be able to apologise later if they have been unreasonable and try to explain to him why the outburst occurred.

As he reaches puberty the development of emotional independence becomes increasingly important. He retains his stable, loving relationship with his parents and from this secure base learns to be a separate individual.

The Parents' Relationship with their Children

Many parents find this a difficult time. The child seems to be growing away from them and they see this as a rejection. If they are clinging or demand too much from him, he will increase the distance between them. If they leave him too much to his own devices he thinks that they are not interested in him and feels hurt and rejected. They have to respect his privacy and his ability to make his own decisions, but still make clear their concern for him.

This is all made much easier if the parents' relationship with each other is thriving and if they have not become emotionally overdependent on the child. They will understand his need for independence and his apparent drawing away from them and not be hurt, if their main emotional ties are to each other. If the parents are hurt and unable to console each other they will feel angry and resentful towards the child and he will feel guilty, angry and resentful in return. This is the basis of many problems which arise between adolescents and their parents. It is the source of much misery and ill health in women approaching middle age, who frequently visit the doctor at this time.

However carefully she has cultivated her own interests and preserved her independence and individuality, any woman with children will have been closely involved with them. They will have absorbed her time and energy, received her love, caused her anxiety. They are more important to her than anything or anyone else except, if she is lucky, her husband. At this stage her marriage may be going through a dull patch. Her husband is very involved with his work and is tired when he comes home. Sex may be infrequent and rather boring, contraception a worry. They have been living together for a long time, working hard and chronically short of money, while the children were at school. In this situation the children may become more important even than the husband and she may find herself imposing intolerable emotional strains on them. She may expect love and support and company and help in the house to a degree which any normal adolescent will resent. If he turns his anger on his mother, she thinks him unloving and ungrateful and their previously happy relationship is soured. Matters deteriorate when she is jealous of his girlfriend. Exactly the same process can happen with a daughter. A sympathetic counsellor may be able to provide some of the support and comfort which the woman should be finding within her marriage and thereby take the strain off the child.

The other major area of conflict concerns the parents' expectation of the child's obedience to them. The natural parents achieve the co-operation of their children not by enforcing obedience but by encouraging the child to want to do what they want. In adolescence he continues to please himself by pleasing them. If obedience has been enforced during his early years and has been grudgingly accepted by him, then he readily rejects it when he reaches adolescence and is no longer so clearly under his parents' control. He is now capable of doing what he wants to do and if that does not happen to be what his parents want, then it is unfortunate.

At this age a father often feels it is his particular responsibility to enforce discipline and comes into open conflict with his son or daughter. He may have extra difficulty in accepting both his daughter's growing sexuality and the threat, as he sees it, to her and to his relationship with

Family Life

her, of boyfriends. The mother is often torn between the children and her husband in this conflict. It is impossible for her not to be involved. However hard she tries, she appears to be taking sides. Often they both think she is against them. She may well have sympathy and understanding for them both but still find the problems difficult to live with and impossible to solve. The stress may bring her to the surgery and if the underlying problem is recognised then it may be possible to help her. She may be able to suggest a compromise between her husband and child. If he stays in and does his homework during the week, he can stay out late on Fridays and Saturdays. He may have the money they would otherwise spend on clothes and other expenses as an allowance to spend himself, provided he makes it cover everything and does not buy cigarettes or alcohol with it. They must allow him a measure of the independence he will soon have totally, if he is to learn how to use it.

Problems with Children's Behaviour

By the time the help of the primary health care team is sought or accepted, family relationships may already be in a poor state. All members of the family may be to some extent emotionally disabled. Their ability to change their behaviour and attitudes, even if they want to, may be limited. In any given situation there may be no choice for an individual as to how he reacts. This can be seen clearly in the sometimes violent behaviour of adolescents, often girls just after puberty, who have suffered early emotional deprivation. They seem to be full of boiling anger and when their control snaps it bursts out, although the final trigger may seem to the amazed observers to have been a trivial matter. This often leads parents and even teachers to wonder whether the child has 'something wrong' with her. 'It is as if she is having a brainstorm.' She often regrets her behaviour afterwards but is powerless to control it. The reaction of the people around her often makes it worse. The same phenomenon can be seen at all ages and in all areas of behaviour. Most adults assume that children are free to decide how to behave and that when they are naughty this is because they have decided to be so. In fact, human behaviour is not as simply explained as this and the only safe assumption is the opposite one. When John is asked why he has stolen from his mother's purse, he answers 'I don't know.' He should be believed because it is almost certainly true. He is unaware of the resentment he has against his mother for preferring (as he thinks) his younger brother. He does not realise that in distributing largesse at school he is trying to buy the friends he cannot make otherwise because of his emotional problems. If he is simply punished for the offence then his problems increase. If he and his parents can be helped to understand what lies behind his behaviour the inevitability of it may lessen. Instead of being angry and preferring the younger brother still more, the mother may be able to show John how much she really does love and value him. His teacher may agree to show greater appreciation of the good in his work rather than harping on his laziness. With love and encouragement he may not need to steal. This does not mean there is no place for reparation in the management of the incident. It may help John to relieve his feelings of guilt if he can repay the money perhaps by helping with errands or car-washing or deductions from his pocket-money. This is not punishment. It is a natural result of his action.

When a small child cries at night he does so because he is hungry, in pain or craves attention. Parents often look upon the first two as reasonable reasons but the third is called naughtiness. The assumption is that the child has woken up and wondered how he might annoy his parents. He has chosen to cry in order to achieve this aim.

In a nearby town recently, a woman was walking with a boy of about ten. He was obviously fed up and lagged behind, dragging his feet. Twice he stumbled and nearly fell over. On the second occasion she turned on him furiously. 'If you do that again I'll hit you so hard! You are just doing it on purpose. That's how you tear your trousers!' It was a ludicrous reaction and might have been funny if it had not been clear that she really meant it.

In every shopping area, mothers can be observed slapping little children because they are crying. They may be crying because they are bored or cold or have fallen down but the mother's reaction is the same. A child may refuse to eat because he is not hungry or to annoy his mother. Either way it is illogical and unhelpful for her to be angry or to try to persuade him to eat. If he wants to annoy her then she should be wondering why and search for ways of making mealtimes happy and relaxed or even abolishing them, if they have become a battlefield. If he is not hungry, then this should be respected. It means that his body is not physiologically prepared to accept food with the high serum insulin, low blood sugar and active digestive secretions which accompany hunger. If a child is repeatedly persuaded to eat to please his mother then he never feels hungry. He is deprived of one of life's greatest pleasures, that of satisfying hunger, and feels permanently nauseated because of his body's unpreparedness for food. He may even regurgitate the food. Many mothers 'force' children between one and a half and four years to eat because they feel they do not eat enough.

Innumerable examples could be given of children's behaviour which appears to be deliberately provocative or disobedient but which in fact has a much more complex explanation. As a general principle, it is helpful if parents can be encouraged to believe that there is an explanation for the child's behaviour even if it is not clear what it is or they do not understand it or cannot accept it. They may then be able to get together with the child to work towards a solution. It is not possible for them, or anyone else, to impose a change in pattern of behaviour on a child.

Family relationships which appear to have been superficially satisfactory while the children were young, sometimes break down when they reach adolescence. It is particularly difficult to help such families. The underlying problems are too deeply-rooted, too long-standing to be easily removed. Attitudes and relationships are too fixed to be much altered. The counsellor has to resist the temptation to blame the parents and show them how it has all come about, how they have been sowing the seeds of disaster since the child was an infant. This can only make matters worse, however true it is. Sometimes the most that can be achieved is for the relationship between the parents and the adolescent or young adult to be saved from total destruction. If it cannot be repaired, at least vestiges of it can be retained to form the foundation of a new relationship in the future. If the bitterest things can be left unsaid, the worst blows unthrown, it may be possible for the child to return, as an adult, and pick up some of the threads.

Few parents achieve perfection in marriage or in bringing up children. There are certain to be problems at many stages along the way. How well they overcome them may depend on the quality and availability of the help they receive. The primary health care team will be only one of the agencies to which parents with problems will turn. If the problems are complex or the team poorly staffed, they may refer them further, perhaps to the child guidance clinic or marriage guidance counsellor, but they will be able to do a great deal themselves to improve the quality of family life for their patients if they have a clear idea of their aims and limitations, keep a sense of humour and are not overambitious.

Note

1. P.E. Daunt, *Comprehensive Values* (Heinemann, London, 1975).

9 MIDDLE AGE

The current Western fashion for early marriage and small families closely spaced means that many women are grandmothers by their early forties and most have a longer period of adult life after their children have left home than before. This can be an exciting time but it also brings problems.

Most women over forty work outside the home, many in full-time jobs. With two incomes and no children to support, money is much more plentiful. If she had some training before she married or while the children were at school, she may have an interesting and well-paid job. If the marriage was well maintained while the children were growing up, it may now gain fresh impetus. The couple are more relaxed and have fewer worries. They have the house to themselves again and are free to make love on Saturday afternoons if they feel like it, a pleasure usually denied to them when there were children at home. They can afford to buy some luxuries, go out more often, take holidays alone. Each has learnt to tolerate the other's weaknesses and irritating habits and to control his own. They have become used to each other without being bored. They still make each other laugh.

If relationships within the family flourished earlier, the middle-aged woman will see her grown up children often and they will enjoy each other's company. She will be a friend, guide and comforter to them and they will be a source of pride, pleasure and friendship to her. Grandchildren will bring particular joy.

Health Problems in Middle Age

Unfortunately not every woman is happy and fulfilled with a satisfying job, exciting marriage and rewarding relationships with her children. For most, the problems of middle age outweigh the advantages. Many of them are unhappy and they form a high proportion of patients attending the surgery. As a group they have a particularly low health quotient and suffer from a high incidence of organic disease, undiagnosable and neurotic illness, affective disorders and simple misery.

A middle-aged woman is likely to be more self-conscious than others about admitting her unhappiness, so that even if she is aware of it as an important factor in her illness she may be reluctant to mention it. She feels ashamed that she is not making a better job of her life, guilty that she is so dissatisfied. There is no spectacular reason for her to be unhappy: so many other people are worse off; it is something she should be able to handle herself but cannot. She feels helpless, frustrated, even trapped.

Many of the systems of the body are the subject of degeneration or simple wear and tear by this time and even the happiest of ideal women is likely to suffer from backache, joint pains, varicose veins, digestive and menstrual problems from time to time. Rheumatoid arthritis commonly starts at this age; carcinoma of the breast is not unusual; everyone is watchful for carcinoma of the cervix; it is important to diagnose and treat hypertension. Almost any symptom, headache, indigestion, menstrual irregularity, change of bowel habit, can be of serious significance. The unhappy woman under stress is more likely to suffer from organic disease and also more likely to develop symptoms of undiagnosable malaise and neurotic symptoms. This poses great difficulties for the primary health care team.

In the present climate most of the patients will in the first instance see the doctor but in the future it may become as usual for a woman to see a different member of the team. Whoever she sees has to be aware of the full range of possible diagnoses and avoid the danger of grasping the first or most obvious one. Even if a correct diagnosis of organic disease is made, the possibility, even likelihood, of accompanying emotional stress should be borne in mind. It is much more difficult to treat a disease successfully in a patient under emotional stress. The response to treatment is likely to be slow, convalescence prolonged and relapse probable. Recovery and rehabilitation are never complete because the underlying unhappiness is still present. The vulnerability to further illness continues. A woman with a low health quotient is more likely to have menorrhagia and to be recommended to have a hysterectomy. She is likely to recover slowly, develop post-operative chest or wound infections and pain. The abdominal and vaginal wounds heal slowly and continue to be tender for many months. She complains of backache, insomnia and fatigue and indeed looks tired. Three months later she is still unable to return to work or tolerate sex. She puts on weight, visibly ages, becomes depressed. If close attention is paid to all her underlying difficulties when she first attends it may be that in time the menorrhagia will resolve and the hysterectomy be unnecessary. The majority of hysterectomies are carried out for menorrhagia, most of them show no evidence of disease. The incidence of post-operative depression is highest in those women in whom the uterus was found to be normal after removal.[1]

This kind of situation where organic disease is present together with general ill health is the most difficult for the doctor because it is so much easier for him to treat the disease and look no further. In some ways it is what the patient wants him to do. She would much rather have an acceptable disease than a shameful emotional problem. It is easier for her to submit to treatment than to work out her difficulties, even with help.

However, it is not in the interests of either patient or doctor for the deeper problems to be ignored even if they are difficult to handle. Even if they can never be completely removed, just to uncover them makes them easier to live with and raises the health quotient a fraction.

Explaining the Deeper Problems

The largest group of middle-aged women attending the surgery are those with symptoms of undiagnosable or benign untreatable disease. One of the commonest is backache. Everyone gets backache from time to time. It is sometimes accompanied by radiological evidence of degeneration but often is not and the symptoms are not directly related to the radiological appearances. It is least likely to be a serious problem in women with a high health quotient who take regular physical exercise. It is a major problem in women with a low health quotient whose muscular tone is poor and general resilience reduced. In them the pain is more severe, lasts longer and is more disabling. It responds less readily to analgesics.

If it is immediately clear that the patient's social and emotional problems are more important than the physical symptom, then it is better to concentrate on those than to waste time investigating the backache but if there is some doubt or the pain is very persistent then it may be useful to do a full blood count, ESR and X-ray even if only to put the doctor's mind at rest and encourage the woman to work on the underlying difficulties.

Headache is another common and sometimes worrying symptom. A careful history and brief examination, including blood pressure and retinoscopy, should make clear whether it is likely to be associated with serious intracranial pathology. If any doubt remains a skull X-ray may help. Even if it is classically migrainous, it should be borne in mind that migraine is more frequent and more severe in someone under stress. The more usual tension headache can be satisfactorily treated only by looking at the whole woman and her circumstances.

Both backache and headache commonly accompany depression. Specific symptoms of even quite severe depression often have to be searched out. It is useful to cultivate a sixth sense, a special alertness for non-verbal signs of depression: a slack, limp look with drooping mouth and shoulders, a beaten expression, dull eyes, difficulty in describing how she feels, talking with an effort. Some women attempt to cover up these signs with a bright, brassy gloss — the classical smiling depression. The eyes often provide a clue: a slightly harassed, vacant, haunted look. She may appear distracted and have difficulty in taking in what is said to her. There is obviously pain but it is not only in her back or her head.

Menopause

Some women sail through the menopause without noticing it. Others are devastated by it. It seems likely that part of the reason for the difference is physiological. Some women rely for oestrogen production almost entirely on their ovaries and as these become less active, the oestrogen supply falls and eventually virtually ceases, whereas others have alternative sites of oestrogen production which continue to function after the menopause. However, this is clearly not the whole story because women with a high health quotient suffer much less from the effects of the menopause than do those with a low one, and those who have previously suffered ill health continue to do so but with greater intensity during the menopause in addition to developing those symptoms specifically related to hormonal changes. It is difficult to distinguish clinically exactly which symptoms are associated with low levels of oestrogen and which to other causes. One reason seems to be that the effect of low oestrogen levels amongst other things is to make a woman more vulnerable to stress than she might otherwise be. When a woman is obviously suffering from the effects of stress it may be impossible to know whether this is because the degree of stress is extreme or whether her resistance is reduced because of oestrogen deficiency or some other cause. Biochemical techniques may make this easier.

The most obvious physiological changes associated with the menopause are those affecting the menstrual cycle. This may suddenly stop without any prior warning or may be erratic for many months or several years before finally disappearing. Sudden amenorrhoea can be worrying in a woman in her forties as it may be due to pregnancy but the older she is the less serious is the likelihood of this. Grossly erratic bleeding with spotting on isolated days or post-coital bleeding should be investigated further at least with vaginal examination and smears and probably with a D & C. Menorrhagia is common and sometimes presents difficult problems. If it is severe, interfering with her activities or making her anaemic and, if this is what she wants, she should be offered hysterectomy, and if it is to be done then it would seem sensible to do it sooner rather than later. However it is a pity to rush into it when the cycle may revert to normal at any time or stop altogether. If she has massive associated problems then it is probably best to postpone hysterectomy for a while, partly because she is a bad candidate at present and her chances of peri-operative and post-operative morbidity may be improved by help with her difficulties, and partly because help with the problems may obviate the need for any interference. The other physiological changes of the menopause are more subtle and effect skin tone and texture, hair and breasts and the state of the mucosa of vulva and vagina.

Hot flushes are the most universal symptom of the menopause but their frequency and severity is extremely variable. They are a good example of a symptom which a woman may want to discuss with a doctor without necessarily having treatment. The natural history of hot flushes is for them to be troublesome for a few weeks or months, then lessen or disappear for a while and reappear later for another spell. There is no way of knowing precisely how they will behave in a particular individual. When this is explained, many women prefer to put up with them for a while and wait to see if they settle down soon on their own without becoming intolerable. She is more likely to be happy to do this if she is assured that she can return for some medication if it gets worse or she changes her mind. The drugs commonly used are tranquillisers, clonidine and oestrogens. There is no rationale for the use of tranquillisers in the treatment of hot flushes unless the woman is exceptionally agitated. Even then they should be used for a few days only while her other problems are being identified. Clonidine seems to help some women but may act only by procrastination so that the symptom disappears naturally while the woman waits for the drug to act.

Hormone replacement therapy does work for this as well as for the relief of other symptoms of oestrogen deficiency. It should not be given to women with a history of thromboembolism, jaundice or breast or genital carcinoma and special care is needed with diabetes and hypertension. The woman should be examined before starting the treatment as for starting an oral contraceptive and should have cervical and posterior fornix smears, blood pressure, examination of the breasts and urine test for sugar. Hormone replacement therapy is probably best given in a cyclical manner with a progestogen added during the second half of the cycle and a tablet-free week in every month. Another important symptom of oestrogen lack is dryness of the vagina and vulva causing dyspareunia and sometimes associated with secondary infection. This is relieved by systemic hormones but local oestrogen in the form of cream or pessaries may be preferable.

Oestrogen deficiency is often associated with demineralisation of bones and with the onset of osteoarthritis. Hormone replacement therapy can prevent these problems but it is doubtful if it is of benefit after they have already developed. If it could be forecast which women were going to develop them, prophylactic treatment could be instituted but this is difficult at present. It is known that women who have a bilateral oophorectomy are more likely to develop osteoporosis and so there is something to be said for giving them routine prophylactic hormone replacement therapy, if the operation was not done for malignant disease.

There is still no general agreement about the possible role of oestrogens in causing carcinoma of the uterus and until this is clarified it seems sensible to limit prescribing to those who clearly need it and not to continue for longer than necessary. An outside limit of three years would be wise.

These are for the most part simple, practical problems. The most difficult aspects of the menopause both for the woman to bear, her family to live with and the primary health care team to help are those related to reduction in resilience, vulnerability to stress and lability of mood. She is more likely to contract infections, have accidents and develop psychiatric illness than earlier in her life or even during the years immediately following.

The Source of Problems in Middle Age

If this reduction in health quotient is associated with oestrogen deficiency then it can be improved by hormone replacement therapy, but is not always and, whether it is or not, help with related problems is still needed. Although the doctor is most likely to have been the first person the woman turned to, he may well not be the best person to help her with her problem. However he will need to understand the range of problems if he is to refer her appropriately to perhaps the community psychiatric nurse, a marriage guidance counsellor or a social worker. The source of her difficulties is likely to be deep-rooted in her early life even though her immediate circumstances are what are causing her unhappiness. To have forged a happy situation for herself in middle age she will have to have been emotionally able-bodied all her life and this will depend upon the quality of mothering and family life she herself received as a child. A high proportion of women had a poor start in this respect and are to some extent emotionally disabled. To expect them to be happy and self-sufficient is like expecting a spastic child to become an athlete, but like the spastic child they may be enabled to improve their performance if they can make the most of the ability they do have and to accept their limitations.

However competent a mother she has been, the growing up of her children, their increasing independence and finally their leaving home will be a sadness to her. There will be a space in her life and feelings which will be hard to fill. If the relationship with the children has not been good then she will see little of them after they leave home and their departure will be more like a total loss, a bereavement. This can start while they are still living at home and can be likened to a terminal illness: a dying relationship. The fact that it is a long drawn out process and there are occasional revivals or sparks of life does not make it any easier to bear.

The one thing which might sustain a woman through this is a happy, supportive marriage but if relationships with children have been poor, it is likely that the family as a whole has been unhappy and the marriage unsettled. If she is still married to the father of the children then they will have been together for a considerable time and their relationship may be dull and stale. If they have run out of conversation, or never had any, sex has become boring and the romance has grown dim, then they may also be unable to offer much in the way of sympathy and comfort to each other. Her husband may find it difficult to appreciate the depth of her misery let alone understand it and may become angry if she tries to explain, thinking that she is in some way blaming him. Whatever her age, he is likely to dismiss all her problems as being part of the menopause and therefore mysterious, incomprehensible and not worthy of consideration. She might be able to revive her flagging spirits if she has an interesting job, but this will depend upon the education and training she has had and on the extent to which she kept up her outside interests and skills during the early years of her marriage. The work available to an unqualified middle-aged woman is mostly boring and poorly paid. If she married young without further education or training after leaving school and devoted all her time and energy to servicing the needs of her family, neglecting her own individuality, friends and interests, she will have great difficulty in finding a satisfactory role for herself now that the family can no longer occupy her individual attention. She feels useless and unwanted and perhaps unloved.

The help a woman most needs will depend on her situation, her attitude to her difficulties and on local factors within the community.

Her emotional problems will need airing to some extent but she may also benefit from practical help. There are considerable advantages in not having a full-time paid job. She will not be so tired, will have time to meet friends and cultivate interests and will be available to visit and if necessary care for her grandchildren. She may be encouraged to find part-time or voluntary work and may still be young enough to benefit from further education or training. An increasing number of middle-aged women take Open University courses or revive an interest in sport.

Any marital difficulties should be studied if possible with the husband as well. Contraception can cause much anxiety. Most women over forty probably should not take an oral contraceptive, the barrier methods are often not acceptable to the patient and intra-uterine contraceptive devices are falling into disfavour with the reputation of a high incidence of pregnancy, pelvic inflammatory disease and menorrhagia. Sterilisation is becoming increasingly popular in this age group. It is unnecessary for any woman to continue with contraception for more than two years after her last period or after she is fifty.

Note

1. D.H. Richards, 'Depression After Hysterectomy', *Lancet*, vol. 2 (1973), p. 430.

10 OLD AGE

The problems of retirement and ageing receive much publicity. The ghettos of some old people's homes and the unbalanced communities of the Costa Geriatrica are often in the news. There are demands for more old people's homes and more hospital beds for the chronic sick. Already the vast majority of patients receiving hospital treatment are over the age of sixty. The problems of the elderly mentally ill are increasing all the time. The problems of the elderly are real and agonising and a serious matter of concern, but this should not be allowed to obscure the fact that old age need not be miserable, lonely and painful — a necessarily evil time to be passed while waiting to die. It can be happy and satisfying, a contented and enjoyable rounding off of life and ultimately an appropriate and helpful preparation for an easeful death. Whatever the circumstances surrounding it, the process of dying is easier in old people. They have a degree of acceptance of it, even of welcome which contrasts sharply with the anguish of those dying young.

Enjoying Old Age

The lessening of the more burdensome responsibilities and tedium of work, and the extra free time which retirement brings, open up exciting possibilities for anyone able to take advantage of them. At last there is time to look around and think, to be peaceful and unhurried. It is possible to see and hear things never noticed before, to have new and uplifting, even exciting experiences, to rediscover old pleasures. Certainly there will be things the old woman cannot do due to physical disability or shortage of money but these face everyone to some extent throughout life. She is likely to be a widow especially if she is very aged, and will have to contend with loneliness and grief, as friends and relatives die, and the prospect of her own death. With help and support, these need not destroy her interest in life and joy in living if she has the qualities needed to make the most of her opportunities. As with the maintenance of health and happiness at any other time of life, success depends upon the personality of the individual, the confidence, the self-respect, the drive. Some people have these qualities in abundance and live life to the full throughout. Most people have them in part but lose them or are unable to use them when times are hard. The stresses and strains of old age are severe and tax the personal reserves of even the most determined. Appropriate help at the right time can enable an old woman to overcome a difficulty, rediscover her ability to live happily and healthily and restore her to the ranks of those who enjoy their old age.

Marriage after retirement can bring particular joy but for some couples, new problems arise and old ones may be magnified. Those who enjoy each other's company and have both shared and separate interests may be happier than they have ever been. They see more of each other but are not together all the time. They continue to interest and amuse each other and provide care, comfort and company, and nursing when necessary, but each retains his own freedom and individuality. The qualities and abilities needed by the widow on her own are equally important to married people in old age. (They will be examined later in this chapter.) The lack of them leads to the problems. If the man's lifelong interest and sole occupation has been his job, then he may be at a loss to fill his time when he stops work. He will become bored and depressed and irritate his wife, being 'always under her feet'. It is interesting how many men like this do not live long past retirement. Their natural drive enables them to resist stresses of all sorts as long as there is something worth doing, but fails them when the future suddenly seems empty. It is a great help if retirement can be approached gradually over a long period. Work can be lighter and hours shorter for several years before official retirement and part-time light work can be continued indefinitely afterwards. This can apply to both sexes and gives them time to learn how to use their leisure and to develop hobbies and interests during late middle life which they can continue into old age. It also raises morale and lessens the feeling of uselessness, of 'being on the scrap heap' which overwhelms some people at this time.

Couples who have been able to share domestic chores throughout their lives and continue to do so seem to enjoy old age more. The old man can have fun cooking and feels less useless if his wife is tired or ill. They can both care for grandchildren and make a welcome refuge for adolescents temporarily at odds with their parents. More and more old people have a car. It is much more use to them if they can both drive it.

Pre-retirement classes are run by some companies and local authorities. Where they are not, they could be instigated or even run by members of the primary health care team. They can encourage the development of new skills such as wood-carving, pottery, tapestry or interests such as music or bird-watching, and provide a meeting place for people to share hopes and fears, ideas and difficulties. They can discuss any aspects of life and ageing, including health, sickness, diet and sex. Personal cleanliness is often neglected by the elderly and upsets their spouses and family. This and a number of other topics can be raised by the health visitor. Other professional experts can be invited to join the discussions.

Many couples continue to derive comfort and pleasure from sexual activity into extreme old age. More than ever it requires love and tolerance, humour, understanding and tenderness. So-called senile vaginitis may affect any woman past the menopause and make intercourse dry and painful. It can be corrected by lubricant creams or hormone replacement, given either locally or systemically depending on the needs of the individual. Many men are unable to achieve or maintain an erection at times, but provided they are not discouraged and continue to try, the capacity usually recovers. Neither they nor their wives should expect too frequent a performance. If full intercourse becomes impossible or uncomfortable then mutual masturbation may provide considerable satisfaction. Just being physically close is a pleasure.

It is extremely important for couples not to be separated in old age and a much greater effort could be made in this respect. Most illness can be treated at home or with a very short admission to a local community hospital under the care of the general practitioner where visiting is easy. Much greater use could be made of nursing homes where both partners could be admitted for a short illness. Even when prolonged illness or permanent severe disability requires continuous nursing care, a couple should still be able to live together in a nursing home or sickbay of an old people's home. All that is needed is greater imagination in planning. The present system of caring for elderly chronic sick people in hospitals is very expensive. The same amount of money could be used differently and with greater humanity and success.

In the meantime, the primary health care team can do a great deal to extend the time elderly couples can stay together in their own homes.

Maintaining Independence

Happy old people are those who retain their independence and enthusiasm for life and who fully occupy their time with activities which interest them. The greater the degree of independence, the easier it is to be happy, but without enthusiasm and interesting occupation, independence cannot on its own make anyone happy. It does not matter whether the occupation is a continuation of paid or voluntary work, an absorbing hobby or the company of other people at clubs or bingo, or a mixture of many activities. What is important is that she has enthusiasm for what she is doing. The ability to do this does not depend on physical health or financial circumstances, although these may limit the choice of activities. It depends upon the personality and previous lifestyle of the woman and her attitude to herself and her situation. A woman, who all her life has retained her self-respect, a consciousness of her own value, a sense of responsibility for her own life, and kept up with her friends and interests, is well equipped to occupy herself in old age. She values the freedom retirement gives her, the opportunity to expand her interests and develop friendships. The one who selflessly devoted herself to her husband and children all her life, denying her own individuality, is less able to occupy her time in an interesting way when their need for her is no longer immediate and obvious. She can find no other role for herself in life. Because the role of the elderly in society is so much less clear than that of the young, they have to be prepared to live life more for its own sake. If by doing so they can maintain their enthusiasm and dignity, their independence and their relationships, they will in fact be making their contribution to society and it will become clearer to them what it is.

This is an area in which all the members of the primary health care team and many other organisations within the community are involved and can work together. The members of the primary health care team are particularly well placed to recognise the need for help when an old woman seems to be in danger of becoming bored and isolated. They also know what activities are available in the community and where there is an opportunity for her to help or visit someone else. They may be able to improve relationships within the family or help her to make a new friend. There are instances of very successful work by a community psychiatric nurse in arranging for a younger woman, who has herself been depressed, to befriend an old one to the mutual benefit of both.

Independence is important in several different aspects of life. They can be grouped under three headings: financial, emotional (family and friends) and physical (health and housing). The members of the primary health care team can be instrumental in the maintenance of independence for an old woman under all these headings. She should have charge of her own money whatever its source and however little it is, but she may need help in budgeting, in accepting that supplementary benefit is not 'charity', and in knowing about and claiming all that she is entitled to.

Emotional Independence

Emotional independence is something everyone needs, but not completely. Love between human beings consists in part of emotional interdependence and to possess total independence would mean to be without loving relationships. On the other hand, too great an emotional dependence on another person destroys love as a relationship. Each partner in a loving relationship should be to some extent emotionally free of the other and able to stand alone. Only then can the relationship thrive. Neither feels leant on or devoured by the other, each feels secure in the other's affection. They need each other equally. It is only on this basis that an elderly woman can get on really well with her family and friends. It is a difficult balance to maintain, the more so because most people do it unconsciously without even being aware of what they are aiming at. It comes most easily to those women who have lived like this all their lives, who have retained their self-respect and personal freedom but even for them it may be more difficult in old age. An old woman is not needed by others in the way that a young mother is needed by her children or a nurse by her patients or even a shop assistant by her customers. Her role is much less easily defined, her contribution to the lives of others more subtle, her purpose in life easier to lose sight of. Even those who know what they are trying to do may be too frail and emotionally battered to carry out their intentions without help and support. A great deal of insight, understanding and even intuition are needed on the part of the helper to identify a woman who is beginning to lose her emotional independence, and to help her back onto her feet again, but it is well worth doing.

The emotionally independent woman has an easy, relaxed relationship with her family and friends, based on mutual love, respect and trust and not on her dependence and their sense of duty. She enjoys the company of her children and grandchildren but does not need it and makes no excessive demands on it. When she is ill they happily nurse her, satisfying their own need to be needed, and she willingly accepts their help, recognising that they gain from giving it. She gives and accepts friendship in the same way, confident that what she gives is as valuable as what she receives. She has no problems with loneliness or social isolation. She is unlikely to develop a depressive illness.

The woman who loses or has never had emotional independence has unsatisfactory relationships with her family and friends. She seems grasping of their time and hard to please. However much they see her or do for her she complains that they neglect her. The relationships are in some way unsatisfying. She seems insatiable because she never gets what she wants: a mutually loving relationship. Bitterness, guilt, anger and resentment poison the atmosphere between the ageing mother and her children. She finds it difficult to make friends and 'keeps herself to herself'. She is an emotional miser. Family and neighbours avoid her.

She has few friends, she becomes socially isolated, lonely and depressed.

Where to Live?

Most old people prefer to live in their own home, but when this is not possible or the family house is too big or far from relatives, it is often helpful to have someone with whom to discuss the alternatives. Often an old woman, recently widowed, is persuaded to move from her home to live with or near a married daughter some distance away. Sometimes this works well but it may be more important for her to stay in the neighbourhood in which she has lived for many years than to be close to her daughter. To leave her home, familiar surroundings and friends would be a second bereavement coming immediately after the first. In this unhappy state of mind she is likely to find it difficult to make new friends and keep up her hobbies and interest in life. Depression is likely to set in and may prove resistant to treatment. A health visitor or social worker may be able to help her to work out what best to do and prevent her from making a hurried decision which she will regret.

Little thought is given to the physical needs of old people when a move to a new home is arranged. People who cannot manage stairs are given first-floor flats and those who cannot walk far find themselves at the top of a hill some distance from the shops. Sometimes a small rearrangement or extra help can enable an elderly woman to continue to live in her old home. She may take a lodger, let part of her house or accept a home help to do housework she can no longer manage. If even this is not possible she should at least always have one room which is hers alone and which contains her own furniture and belongings and for the care of which she is responsible.

Preventing Disability

The maintenance of physical independence in terms of health depends on the prevention of disability and the treatment of symptoms. The prevention of disability in elderly women is a most important aspect of the work of the whole primary health care team and one which is usually neglected. It has to start during youth and middle life with anti-smoking propaganda, the treatment of hypertension, which reduces the number of strokes, and the treatment of obesity, which is a major immobilising factor in the elderly. There is very little which can be done to prevent the wear and tear on joints which become swollen, stiff and painful with age and osteoarthritis, but a thin old woman with this problem will be able to continue to be active while a fat one will be immobilised. The same principle applies to ischaemic heart disease and chronic bronchitis. It is very hard for an old woman, set in her dietary habits and relatively inactive, to lose weight, but she may be able to keep slim if that is how she starts her retirement. Few women take any exercise once they have left school but those who do and who keep it up into old age are at a great advantage. They find it easier to keep their weight down and feel fitter, more energetic and supple. Swimming is one of the best forms of exercise because it does not damage joints which may already be worn, but any form is better than none. Old people who have never taken any exercise may be persuaded to join a keep-fit or yoga class if they are sure others of their own age will be there. It may be possible to arrange a special group in an over-60s club.

The close relationship between physical fitness and state of mind is even more obvious in old age than at other times of life. True depressive illness is common in the elderly, and it is disabling, but a greater problem is a chronic low-grade misery short of depression which afflicts many people and lowers their resistance to disease and stresses of all sorts. It destroys the woman's independence at all levels in a much more devastating way than any purely physical disability. With no enthusiasm for life, she goes out less, neglects friendships and interesting activities. She becomes unable to cope with minor illness and aches and pains which someone else might ignore. She allows them to incapacitate her more than they need and her joints stiffen. She in fact becomes less mobile and more likely to develop infections, put on weight and become really depressed. If this tendency can be recognised at an early stage when the woman is still physically fit, it may be possible to stimulate her interest in life and halt her downward slide. She may be willing to help a disabled neighbour, or raise money for the church or babysit for a harassed mother, even if she feels unable to join a club or invite a neighbour in at first. The primary health care team is ideally situated to identify the need and administer what in effect is true prophylactic treatment.

The prevention of disability in the elderly depends on recognising at an early stage factors which may lead to problems later. The woman may not herself be concerned about anything and not actively seeking help. It is therefore necessary for the primary health care team to make sure that all elderly people are seen at regular intervals. This has to be carefully planned. It is no use the doctor popping in once a month for a social chat if he fails to discover that she has a painful corn which prevents her going out or such poor lighting that she thinks her vision has deteriorated and has given up embroidery which was her main interest. She is unlikely to mention a lump in the breast over tea, let

Old Age

alone vaginal bleeding. It is better for the health visitor to call once a year with a check list so that nothing is missed and the woman has an opportunity to complain about her inefficient heating or shortness of breath.

The Function of the Primary Health Care Team

Each team will want to make its own list and own arrangements about who should see which people. Some will be in contact already. If the nurse sees the woman every three months at the surgery for her injection of cytamen, then she can complete the questionnaire when it is due. If the doctor visits when she has a fall, then he can do it. It is important to make sure no one is missed and that something is done when potential problems are identified.

The sort of questions which are useful to ask are set out below, but the interviewer must be watching for readiness on the part of the woman to elaborate on any point. It may be that no question on the list reveals her particular problem except in a roundabout way. Some questions seem to cover the same ground as others, but this can be useful and one may reveal a problem when another does not. Questions can be omitted if they are obviously irrelevant. The questionnaire should be in a form which can be filed in the medical records. It is helpful if it can first be completed on retirement or by the age of seventy and then annually.

Housing

Does she need help with decorations, repairs, garden, furnishing, housework?
Is the home adequately heated and well lit, especially where she sits and on stairs?
Are there any trailing cables, loose rugs, unguarded or dangerous heaters?
Does she need any special aids?
Are there any problems, e.g. with stairs or position of home?

Social

Is she keeping up with family, friends, neighbours, clubs?
Does she need help with transport to do so?
Does she need a telephone?
Who does she see every day/occasionally?
Is she lonely?
Are there any problems?
Can she do her own shopping, housework, cooking?
Can she wash, dress and feed herself?

Is there anything she would like to do but cannot?

Financial

Is she claiming all that she is entitled to, e.g. help with fuel costs, rent and rate rebate, supplementary benefit?
Is she paying for anything she need not, e.g. bus fares when pass is available, income tax?

Health

Is she happy?
Has she any worries or fears?
Does she think about dying?
Does she go out? If not, why not?
How far can she walk?
Does she feel well?
Has she any symptoms new or old? Ask specifically about breast lumps, vaginal and rectal bleeding, breathlessness, chest pain, oedema, dysuria, stress, incontinence, frequency of micturition, trouble with feet, feeling cold, tired, slowed up.
Are all her bodily functions normal? Run through them.
Are her hearing and vision normal?
Is she taking any medicines? If so, is she taking them correctly? Does she need them? Does she want them/understand them?
Can she get to the surgery? If not, could she if transport were provided?

This can be an opportunity to discuss general problems, hopes, fears, plans and anxieties about members of the family. There should be an opportunity to talk about dying. She may welcome this. It is something which may be on her mind but which she cannot discuss with anyone else. Most old people are not afraid of death but fear illness and especially helplessness and total physical dependency and the process of dying. It may help for the vicar to call.

Whilst prevention of disease and disability are far more effective than treatment, nevertheless there are a number of measures which can be taken to alleviate the problems of established disability. All the members of the team may be involved.

Alleviating Established Disabilities

Chiropody, walking aids, a wheelchair and special aids around the home can all help to improve mobility. A hearing aid or speech therapy following a stroke can help the woman's ability to communicate. Expert help with incontinence or a colostomy can transform the life of an old person. A home help, meals on wheels and regular visits from the bathing attendant can be used for short-term problems as well as with long-standing ones. A magnifying-glass, good lighting or a talking book may help the partially sighted or blind.

Some diseases in old age respond well to treatment. Heart failure, hypothyroidism, chest infections and Parkinson's disease are particularly rewarding. Less common, and therefore more likely to be missed, are heart block, with Stokes Adams attacks causing falls, and hyperthyroidism, which is often in its 'forme fruste' in the elderly and presents with atrial fibrillation and angina or loss of weight without other obvious signs or symptoms. Accuracy and completeness of diagnosis are as important as in the young, but sometimes more difficult, and require a high degree of alertness on the part of the doctor. It is particularly common to find more than one disease in an old person and it is therefore necessary to look beyond the most obvious diagnosis. Angina is due to ischaemic heart disease, but if the patient is anaemic or thyrotoxic one of these may be the immediate precipitating cause. Anaemia may also produce the symptoms of intermittent claudication although the underlying cause is peripheral vascular disease.

Many people with cough and dyspnoea come to the doctor asking for 'something for the bronchitis'. If the doctor accepts the patient's diagnosis he will miss a number of cases of left ventricular failure which might have responded well to treatment. When the differential diagnosis really is difficult, there is no harm in giving a diuretic and an antibiotic.

Using Hospital Facilities

In the care of the elderly it is especially useful to have close links with the local hospital. Most elderly people are afraid of hospitals. They find attendance at outpatient clinics exhausting and confusing and are demoralised, disorientated and frightened by admission as an inpatient. As far as possible, old people should have investigations and treatment at home. For instance, if the general practitioner has open access to laboratory and X-ray facilities, it will hardly ever be necessary to refer or admit patients to hospital for the investigation of anaemia. A full blood picture and chemistry, faecal occult blood and urinalysis are easily carried out at the surgery and patient's home by the nurse and the samples sent to the laboratory. There is usually someone who can help with transport for a chest X-ray or even barium studies if these are necessary. Bone marrow samples can be taken as an outpatient.

An old person with hyperthyroidism can be investigated by the general practitioner and treated with radioactive iodine at one single outpatient visit. No hospital follow-up is necessary as the primary health care team can watch for, investigate and treat the hypothyroidism which eventually develops. In fact it can do this more efficiently than can the hospital. No one can say within a number of years when the hypothyroidism will develop. When it does, the patient may deteriorate quite quickly, certainly within three months. If she is attending hospital outpatients once a year or even at six-monthly intervals, she may have had to attend for a very long time before the need is apparent and then may have suffered for many months before being treated. She can see the nurse at the surgery for a brief word every three months and have her weight and pulse rate checked. Her thyroid function tests can be done annually or whenever there is any doubt. This involves her in no distress or expense and is cheaper for the health service.

Diabetes is another condition which should not involve regular attendance at a hospital apart from occasional appointments at an eye clinic for retinoscopy. Again, open access to the laboratory is important as also is an easy relationship with a consultant who can be asked about particular problems without taking over the care of the patient. A plan for the care of diabetes is useful and the tasks are shared within the primary health care team. The nurse can ensure that the diet is adhered to, the urine tested and the results satisfactory, the weight steady and blood sugar checked at intervals agreed with the doctor. The receptionist may be the one to arrange chiropody if there is no chiropodist within the team, and transport if necessary for this and for the routine chest X-ray.

If the common combination of osteoarthritis and obesity form the disability, an energetic plan to lose weight, relieve pain and increase mobility could involve dietician, doctor and physiotherapist. The dietician may in fact be a nurse or health visitor who contacts the district dietician for advice if she needs it. A physiotherapist who would treat people in their homes or at a health centre or even in groups in a community centre would be a great help. The social worker may be needed to provide special aids in the home.

Medication and the Elderly

All medication in the elderly should be kept as simple and as sensible as possible. It often happens that a new drug is introduced and added on to what the patient was previously taking. It is not unusual for an old woman to be taking aspirin, indomethacin and ibuprofen from her doctor as well as a proprietary analgesic which she buys herself. Many take valium three times a day and mogadon at night despite the fact

Old Age

that both are chemically almost identical and equally long-acting. Some may be found to be taking three different diuretics. Many drugs traditionally given in divided doses are equally effective if given once a day. These include thyroxine, tranquillisers, anti-depressants and β-blockers. Many anti-rheumatics can be given effectively once a day at night or at most morning and night. It is very easy for modern drugs to do more harm than good and there is evidence that this often happens. It is the doctor's responsibility to see that his prescribing is safe and benefits the patient, but the whole team can help to ensure that patients understand about drugs, take them correctly and that side-effects do not pass unnoticed. Elderly people taking diuretics may develop hypokaloemia which makes them extra sensitive to digitalis overdosage, and also postural hypotension, causing faints and falls. Tranquillisers and hypnotics have disastrous effects on some old people, making them confused or even demented.

The doctor should make clear in his notes all the drugs the patient should be taking including both those he gave her previously and which should be continued as well as those he has just prescribed. Instruction for taking medicines should be written out clearly on a card or sheet of paper as well as on each bottle. It might look like this:

Mrs Mary Smith	21 October 1979
Lasix tablets (white) 40 mgm (for breathlessness and swelling of the ankles)	one each morning
Digoxin tablets (pale blue) 0.0625 mgm (steady the heart)	one each morning except Sundays
Soluble aspirin tablets (white) 300 mg (for pain from arthritis)	two after breakfast two after midday meal two after tea two at bedtime
TNT tablets (white) 300 mg	one under the tongue for pain in chest

Stop the aspirin if you develop indigestion or a tummy upset.
Continue the Lasix even if the breathing and swollen ankles improve.

It is most helpful if the patient can see the nurse occasionally after she has seen the doctor or for the nurse to visit her at home the next day and go through her medication with her. Again, a checklist is useful:

Is she taking any medicines other than those prescribed?
Is she taking only those recently prescribed or has she some left over from a previous time?
Does she understand what each one is for and when and how to take it?
Can she read the instructions on the label/sheet of paper?
Does she need and want all the medicines she is taking?
Does she realise which, if any, she should continue to take even if she feels better and loses the symptom for which it was prescribed (e.g. diuretics for left ventricular failure)?
Has she any symptoms which might be due to side-effects of a drug?

Where to Care for the Elderly

On the whole, old people are more likely to recover, and recover more quickly, from an illness treated at home than one treated in hospital. Many expect to die if they are admitted to hospital, and stop fighting. Some, previously alert, become disorientated in the strange surroundings. Others merely dislike the hospital intensely — the strange people, food, bed and everything about it. All are frightened and being frightened impedes recovery. Quite apart from recovery, most people prefer to die at home. The ensuing grief is easier for the spouse and the rest of the family. The whole business of death is more dignified.

It is therefore to everyone's benefit for old people who are ill to be nursed at home if this is at all possible. From the purely medical point of view of treating the illness, it nearly always is possible. Difficulties arise in the provision of general care and nursing. The whole primary health care team may be needed to carry this out.

The main problem arises when the patient is too weak, too confused or too frightened to be left alone. If she lives with one of her children or if her husband is fit, then help will be needed for only part of the time, and perhaps at night, but if she lives alone, the arrangements have to be more comprehensive. Part of the job of the primary health care team is to co-ordinate members of the family, friends and local care group or other community organisation so that someone can be with the patient for as much of the time as possible and provide normal non-nursing care and company. If this is not quite enough, then in most places the area health authority will provide a certain amount of help, especially at night. Most communities contain plenty of people willing and able to help with this sort of service. If the primary health care team is active and has well-established links with local organisations, then help is always at hand.

The Care of the Dying

If there are doubts about whether the patient will recover, or if she is clearly going to die, the doctor should explain this to those caring for her. Many people are nervous of caring for the sick in case they should do something wrong with disastrous results. They can face the idea that the patient may die if they are prepared first, have the opportunity to talk about it and know what they should do if it happens. Intense fear of death and the dying is a modern phenomenon brought about partly by removing terminal care from the community where it belongs and shrouding it in mystery in hospitals, and partly by the energy with which the medical profession appears to fight death and the diseases which cause it. This is also responsible for the universal terror of cancer which is illogical, as it is usually a more comfortable thing to die from than, for instance, chronic bronchitis, heart disease or a stroke. If dying could be accepted back into the community as a natural experience, the only one, apart from birth, to be shared by everyone, then some of its fearfulness might be removed. This would help the living as well as the dying.

The care of the dying at home is very much a community as well as a primary health care team effort. The ease with which the patient dies may depend more upon the comfortable words of the vicar than on the doctor's drugs. In fact the amount of drugs necessary to relieve pain and other discomforts are found to be less if the patient has peace of mind. The doctor needs to make full use of this knowledge in treating his patient and will also find it helpful to listen carefully to what the patient's attendants have to say. They may be able to give a more accurate account of her needs and symptoms than she herself can or is willing to do. She may put on a brave face for the doctor and be unwilling to admit that his treatment is failing her. Nurses in particular are helpful in this respect. They have a much more intimate knowledge of the effect of drugs in terminal care than has the doctor. This knowledge is based on close personal observation and experience of other patients as well as this one, and the doctor should listen carefully to the nurse's opinion about what drug might benefit the patient. If he rejects her advice, then he should tell her why and explain why he is choosing the régime he is, so that he has her enthusiastic support and co-operation in administering it. Only then are the best results possible.

The presence of members of the family at the bedside of someone who is dying is a great comfort, but it can also have an inhibiting effect on conversation between the patient and the doctor or other professional visitor. The patient may want to talk about his condition and about the future. He may know he is dying and want to share this knowledge and his feelings about it. Relatives often find this painful and embarrassing and it is a help if the patient can be seen alone at least on some occasions. He then may be encouraged to share his feelings at least with his wife. It is extraordinary that a couple who have shared their whole lives and never hidden anything from each other should be unable to talk about the most important event in their lives and one which they have always known would happen. The patient must remain the arbiter of how much if anything he is to discuss and with whom, but the opportunities should be made for him. He can then decide how to use them.

Grief

However well managed the terminal illness, however much the death was to be expected, even welcomed, those left behind grieve. It is a necessary process and one which must be gone through if the threads of life are to be picked up again. The formalities of the funeral rites seem to help and the loss of an accepted period of mourning is a disadvantage of modern society. While there may be much attention paid to the widow by the family immediately after the death of her husband, she is likely to need other help and support soon after. She needs help to live through her grief and not succumb to it, to learn to live with the feelings of loss and guilt and regret which crowd in on her, and in time to look ahead and plan her own future.

Relatives often try to stop the widow grieving, to cheer her up, take her mind off her grief. They may ask the doctor for tranquillisers or hypnotics for her. These probably do little harm for a few days but there is no evidence that they really help and it is possible that they interfere with or at least delay the necessary full expression of grief. It really is important for the widow not to continue to take them after the first few days because they then have a depressing and slowing effect which clearly does impede her recovery.

The love, friendship and support of the community, including the members of the primary health care team, are what she most needs. The provision of these is true preventive medicine. The woman's future health depends on the successful outcome of this period of her life.

11 DEPRESSION AND ANXIETY

Depression

The term 'depression' is used widely and loosely to describe any degree of lowered spirits from the mildest to the most severe. It is experienced by every woman at some time in her life following bereavement, illness or a setback in personal relationships. It is inextricably linked with the concept of health and well being which form the subject of this book and is mentioned in every other chapter. It is such a widespread and massive problem that it merits separate consideration as well as the many passing references it receives. Depression is a part of normal human experience. It becomes a problem, for which help from a doctor or other member of the primary health care team may be sought, when it seems to the sufferer, or her family, that the reaction is out of proportion to the precipitating cause. The condition then becomes a neurotic depressive illness. It is usually taught that depressive psychosis is a completely separate condition occurring in a different type of predisposed person and with a totally different set of clinical features. Whilst it is true that it is possible to find people at either end of the spectrum between neurotic and psychotic depression, it is also clear that there is an area of overlap where the distinction is not so clear.

This chapter deals mainly with neurotic reactive depression. It develops in response to stress and is an extension of a normal process beyond the accepted bounds of normality. Exactly where these bounds lie will depend on the outlook of the individual and her family. What is accepted as normal varies widely and seems to depend partly on social class. Working-class women are more often prepared to accept a degree of chronic depression than those from the middle class.

The Incidence of Depression

There is also a great variation in individual susceptibility to depression. Some people are clearly more vulnerable than others. A tendency to develop depression often runs in families but it is difficult to determine to what extent this is a genetic effect and how much it is due to environmental influences. It seems likely that inherited personality characteristics play some part in the ability of the individual to resist the development of depression, but previous experience, especially in early life, and the present situation are the most important factors. It is often found in women with a low health quotient.

Depression in children is common. It is associated with difficulties, most often emotional, which the child does not understand and cannot sort out. In a young child the commonest source of problems is her relationship with her mother and siblings. She may feel angry and resentful and unable to control her own behaviour. This helplessness later leads to a belief that she is not responsible for her own behaviour and this may be carried into adult life. To be able to resist depression, everyone needs to have confidence in her ability to control her own behaviour and influence what happens to her. If she believes that she is buffeted by external forces beyond her power to resist or alter, this will in fact become true. In this situation difficulties are not overcome, they are succumbed to, and depression follows. Social helplessness is often blamed on the welfare state but it seems more likely to be the result of poor early conditioning and emotional disability. Most people would rather not be dependent either on each other or on the state but many do not have an alternative which they are capable of using.

Unfortunately those who are particularly at risk of developing depression as a result of a deprived childhood are also those most likely to find themselves in situations which increase the risk still further. A woman who finds it difficult to form relationships with other adults, whether her husband or friends, and who cannot communicate easily with them, will fail to derive the help and support which might have enabled her to live through the stressful period without becoming depressed. A woman who does not have a mutually supportive relationship with her husband, or who is socially isolated, is more likely to become depressed than one who has. However caring her husband, if he is inarticulate or mystified by her feelings, he will be of little help to her. Those with several children under school age are particularly vulnerable. Those who work outside the home may get overtired but seem less likely to suffer a depressive illness.[1] This is partly due to contact with other people but also to the satisfaction of doing paid work.

Women approaching middle age are particularly susceptible to depression. This is only indirectly associated with the impending menopause and is not the result of hormonal imbalance or deficiency. It is most likely to affect the woman whose whole purpose in life was to be a wife and mother and make a home for her family. Her need to be needed is paramount but as the children grow up she feels less and less necessary. Her relationships with her children are likely to deteriorate if she depends on them for company. She may have no friends of her own age, no other interests and no training for work outside the home, or lack confidence to seek it. Her marriage is unlikely to provide her with all the interest and fulfilment she needs. Her husband cannot be everything to her nor she to him. Her looks are deteriorating. If, while the children were growing up, she neglected her own apparently selfish interests, gave up her hobbies, lost contact with friends, let her mind vegetate, she will be ill equipped to cope with the loneliness, isolation and uselessness of the life to which she is now committed.

This is a very difficult situation to remedy. She is likely to lack confidence, initiative and the ability to make good relationships, or she would not find herself in this position. She herself is the only one who can alter her circumstances and yet she is probably unable to do so.

The Symptoms of Depression

The symptoms of depression as presented to the doctor are many and varied. Very often they are cloaked in physical symptoms. A woman may complain of fatigue or headache which she may or may not recognise as being due to depression. Another may want help with depression but feel it necessary to present the doctor with an invented or exaggerated physical complaint. Depression affects every aspect of a woman's life, how she functions as well as how she feels. What is brought to the doctor as 'the problem' will vary with her intelligence, social class, upbringing and her relationship with him. Whether she volunteers the information or whether the doctor finds out by questioning her, if she is depressed she will suffer from a persistent feeling of tiredness which is usually present when she first wakes in the morning. She will lack interest and drive and will find difficulty in getting through her work. She may complain of a reduced appetite but in fact be eating more and gaining weight without enjoying her food. She is irritable with her children. She does not bother with her appearance and yet complains that she 'looks a mess'. She is likely to complain of sleeping badly, by which she means fitfully, but falls asleep during the day or evening, and has difficulty waking in the morning. The depression will probably continue all day with no diurnal variation. She may say she 'cannot stand it' and wants to 'get away from everything'.

Backache, headache, facial pain, chest pain, vulvitis, digestive problems, menstrual irregularities and an increased susceptibility to accidents and infection often accompany depression. The severity of the symptoms as described by the patient depends on the rapidity of the onset of the illness. If she has been chronically depressed for a long time then an increase in her symptoms may not seem very dramatic, whereas if the depression is recent and sudden, the same degree of disability will be more impressive. Stress can be lifelong and continuous, such as results from living with an alcoholic husband or handicapped child; intermittent, as might be associated with financial problems or crime; or temporary, as might happen following an accident, illness or bereavement. Whatever the type of stress which precipitates a depressive illness, the way the illness presents and the course it takes will depend on the woman's previous personality and state of mind and on the quality of her relationships and lifestyle. One of the characteristics of a neurotically depressed woman is her inability to view minor symptoms with a sense of proportion. Her susceptibility to organic disease is increased but the intensity with which she feels the symptoms is also increased. A symptom may even continue after the organic cause has clearly resolved. It is then a purely neurotic symptom.

This is a difficult situation for a doctor to sort out. He is irritated with the woman for having a neurotic illness in the first place, but he is well aware of the dangers of dismissing all her symptoms as neurotic and nervous since he may miss organic disease, the diagnosis of which is his *raison d'être*. Her exaggeration of her symptoms, even if unconscious, makes the diagnosis of organic disease more difficult and she may deliberately overstate the symptoms to impress him that she is not being neurotic this time. Resentment builds up quickly on both sides. The only way of dealing with this is for the doctor constantly to remind himself of the interaction and his own part in it. If he is aware of what is going on as it happens he may be able to minimise the worst effects.

Very often the precipitating cause is hard to find. It may be a chronic dissatisfaction with the quality of life. Doctors need to have a high degree of insight to understand what it is like for a woman to live in a modern 'little box' with a nuclear family, the only other adult member of which is away most of the time. She has to be highly self-sufficient to be satisfied and contented with no one but small children for company and nothing but the endless drudgery of housework to do. She may appear to be fortunate in having a loving husband, a nice home, beautiful healthy children. This only heightens the guilt which so often accompanies and exacerbates depression. She clearly should not be depressed. She has nothing to be depressed about but her life consists of getting through each day waiting to start living. It is like moving along in a queue without knowing how long it is or what is at the end.

It is when neurotic depression becomes severe that it approaches the area of overlap with psychotic depression. The characteristics of this include early waking, loss of appetite, constipation, amenorrhoea, loss of weight, loss of libido, loss of concentration, intense anxiety and ideas of suicide all of which are also found in patients with severe, reactive, neurotic depression. Puerperal depression is often severe and sometimes clearly psychotic.

During and after the menopause most women experience increased emotional lability. There is a reduced tolerance of normal stresses which the woman might previously have taken in her stride. She is more irritable and likely to snap at members of the family. Husbands and grown-up children are usually surprisingly tolerant of this situation especially if previous family relationships were good and the problem is intermittent and does not continue for too long. A small proportion of women suffer a menopausal depressive illness similar to the involutional melancholia which also occurs in men and has become an unfashionable diagnosis. It may be severe and require drug treatment or admission to hospital.

Depression in Old Age

This is generally considered to be related to ill health, poverty, disability and bereavement, and of course these are very important factors especially in extreme old age. However, it is surprising how many poor, disabled, bereaved old women have a high health quotient and do not get depressed. Their previous personality and ability to socialise seem to be the most important factors. If they were among the group who felt cast off and useless in middle age, and if they failed to resolve that situation by finding new friends and interests, then their old age is likely to be dull, lonely and unhappy.

Disability in old age includes degenerative disease of joints and it needs courage and determination to continue to be cheerful and active in the face of pain and stiffness. Many old people have these qualities in abundance but they are lost quickly in depression. Once depressed, the old woman becomes more disabled by any other condition from which she may suffer. She is poor company and so family and friends avoid her. She lacks initiative to go out and attend clubs or ask neighbours round and progressively becomes more lonely and isolated.

The Treatment of Depression

There is no place for drugs in the treatment of the vast majority of women suffering from mild to moderate depression. In fact it seems likely that they often make the condition worse. Although she may complain of tension, irritability and difficulty in sleeping, tranquillisers and hypnotics seem to have a sedative and depressing effect without relieving the other symptoms. They make the woman feel more tired than ever, tiredness already being one of her main problems. She will be less efficient in organising her work and her family and this will add to her other difficulties. If hypnotics must be used they should be short acting, not of the barbiturate or benzadiazipine groups and used for a few days only.

Avoiding Drug Treatment

In fact if the alternatives are clearly explained, most women will choose not to take drugs. The reason they are so often prescribed is that few doctors offer their patients a choice of treatments. It is quicker to write a prescription than to explain the alternatives.

The aim of treatment should be to improve the woman's situation and increase her understanding and resilience. Most doctors have not time or skill to do this themselves. With the increasing development of the primary health care team, the inclusion of community psychiatric nurses and social workers and improvement of links with churches, care groups and other voluntary organisations, this situation could change. The doctor will no longer have to offer frequent and repeated long interviews with himself as one of the alternatives unless he feels able and willing to do so. Health visitors, social workers, community psychiatric nurses and voluntary workers such as marriage guidance counsellors should all be available depending on the type of problem and the patient's preference. Already, in areas where community psychiatric nurses or social workers are well established, some patients, who recognise their symptoms, refer themselves directly to these workers, bypassing the doctor altogether, and of course this is what churches have been doing for centuries.

Another reason why drug treatment is unhelpful is because it lessens the determination of the patient, her family and the members of the primary health care team to work at improving the underlying situation. It has often been observed that the person who presents at the surgery for treatment is not the most disturbed member of a family nor the one most needing help. If the doctor prescribes for a depressed woman, whether a placebo or pharmacologically active drug, both he and the patient will then wait for it to take effect. No work will be done on understanding and resolving the underlying problems. Even if she does obtain temporary relief from taking the medicine, the situation continues and the symptoms will recur. Her alcoholic or gambling husband or disturbed child will continue unrecognised and unhelped and she will not even be receiving the support and sympathy she needs to carry on.

Even if the problems arise entirely from her own inadequacy, it is likely that she and the family will benefit from help and support of some sort. Many doctors feel discouraged when treating neurotically depressed women. It is so very unrewarding when they never seem to make any progress and return again and again, with yet another problem. However, there is a great opportunity for community psychiatric nurses and social workers to work with these women and their families to prevent breakdown of the marriage and problems for the children. It may be that counselling in marital problems or help to find a playgroup at an early stage in the development of difficulties will avert serious disintegration of family relationships, marital breakdown or battered children. If every depressed woman were looked on as a warning signal of risk for or problems in her family and followed up, useful work might be done in preventing future problems. Exactly the same principle applies to the follow-up of those admitted to hospital for drug overdosage. The vast majority of such people are not truly suicidal but immature, inadequate or neurotically depressed. This is recognised in the hospital and they are discharged as soon as possible. It is often said that 'she is just attention-seeking' as if this alone is a reason for firmly ignoring her. Even those who admit that it may be a 'cry for help' seldom offer the help or suggest where she might find it. These women, too, should be followed up by an appropriate member of the primary health care team to see if anything more can be done.

Drug Treatment

When depression is severe with early waking, marked lack of interest, loss of concentration, flatness of affect, withdrawal, intense feelings of worthlessness and suicidal thoughts and any of the physical symptoms previously mentioned, drug treatment is useful. It is usually best to give a tricyclic anti-depressant on its own as the addition of a tranquilliser only adds to the sedative side-effects. If there is intense anxiety as well, a tranquilliser may be useful. A course of treatment should be planned and outlined to the patient. There is an initial adjustment period of 3-6 weeks during which the woman is likely to experience side-effects such as drowsiness, blurred vision and a dry mouth. She should be warned of this and reassured that these symptoms will gradually lessen as time passes. She should also be warned that she is unlikely to notice any benefit from the treatment for at least two weeks. If these warnings are not given, she is unlikely to continue to take the drug and her despair will increase at the apparent failure of the treatment.

The drug is best given in a single dose of not less than 75 mg at night but may be split into 25 mg in the morning and the rest at night. If the patient finds the initial side-effects intolerable she can start on a lower dose and increase it gradually. The next phase in the treatment is stabilisation. Her mood will have improved but she will be emotionally frail and should continue to take the full dose of the drug unless side-effects are a problem. This should last 4-8 weeks depending on her previous history, family situation and degree of recovery. The third and last phase of the treatment is reduction of the dose. This should be done gradually. A reduction of 10 mg every one or two weeks is about right, the whole process taking 6-12 weeks. The entire course of treatment will have taken anything from three months to a year. It should be accompanied by a thorough examination by the patient and her therapist, doctor or psychiatric nurse, of the situation which precipitated the depression, and considerable work may have to be done in preventing damage to the family and relapse in the future. If these things are not done, the treatment will have been a waste of time, like going on a crash diet to lose weight and returning to the original eating habits afterwards.

How the supervision of this long course of treatment is conducted will depend on the personnel available. A combination of a doctor and community psychiatric nurse is ideal with help from other agencies if the social circumstances require it.

Relapse is common during the few months after the end of a course of treatment and it is useful for one of the therapists to see the patient at intervals for at least six months to watch for early symptoms and signs of relapse. Anti-depressant drugs must be used with great caution in the elderly as the dose is difficult to gauge and side-effects common. It is also important not to allow old people to take either anti-depressants or tranquillisers for long periods. They may become confused and depressed or even demented as a result. If they do, the dose is often increased, making matters worse. Even quite a small dose, say 10 mg of benzodiazipine at night, can make an old woman aggressive, confused and depressed. The symptoms vanish when the drug is stopped.

As with all other depressed patients, the treatment should be aimed at improving her situation and outlook.

Hospital Treatment

It is not often necessary to admit patients with depression to hospital. However, if the depression is severe with serious risk of suicide or harm to a child, for instance in the puerperium, or if there is no available support from the family or community, then it may be unavoidable. It is essential that the patient receives proper follow-up care from the primary health care team after discharge from hospital. The better the links between the hospital and primary health care team, the easier this will be. For instance, it may be possible for the community psychiatric nurse to visit the patient in hospital and build up a relationship before she is discharged. The patient can be helped by short visits home with support from the community psychiatric nurse. If the woman has a young baby, the baby should be admitted with her and the health visitor enabled to visit them both in hospital.

If depression is treated with energy, enthusiasm and optimism it is more likely to recover and will be less of a burden to the patient, her family, the primary health care team and the community as a whole.

Anxiety

Like depression, anxiety is a well-recognised, normal response to certain types of stress. When the stress is sudden and external, the response is called fear. When it is long-lasting and abstract or spontaneous, it is known as worry or anxiety. Only when the response is exaggerated, occurring without recognisable cause or is out of proportion to the degree of stress does the condition constitute a neurotic illness for which help may be sought. It is a form of breakdown similar in aetiology to depression and many of the same factors are important. Chronic anxiety usually accompanies a low health quotient.

The Symptoms of Anxiety

The symptoms of pathological anxiety are exactly the same as those of physiological fear. They include all the results of increased activity of the sympathetic nervous system associated with the fight/flight response. The symptoms may be present in any number and combination, and one may predominate or several appear of equal importance.

An anxious person may have a tachycardia with palpitations, increased sweating, anorexia, diarrhoea, frequency of micturition and a dry mouth. The respiratory rate may be increased and many anxious people complain of a feeling that they cannot take a deep breath or are unable to fill their lungs fully.

A woman may come to her doctor complaining of feeling anxious or specifically of one of the symptoms. She may appear tense and restless, wringing her hands and have dilated pupils and a tremor. Many of the symptoms of anxiety also occur as part of organic diseases and this may make the diagnosis difficult. A woman with palpitations due to an organic cause may become anxious as a result of worrying about it. One with palpitations due to anxiety may think they are due to an organic cause and become more anxious. Both will seem anxious to the doctor.

Anxiety also heightens the individual's awareness of the many minor discomforts which assail the human body every day. An attack of indigestion which might normally be ignored feels much more intense and assumes fearful significance, twinges of muscular pain are severe and incapacitating.

Depression often accompanies anxiety and when the two occur together, unilateral facial pain, chest pain and low backache are particularly common and troublesome symptoms.

The Treatment of Anxiety

The doctor first has to make sure that there is no organic disease underlying the patient's complaint. This is important to reassure both the patient and the doctor and to enable work on the anxiety to go ahead. Treatment of any organic disease is probably of secondary importance but there are some conditions such as hyperthyroidism which may be confused with an anxiety state and which are well worth treating. The unilateral facial pain of the woman with a combined depression-anxiety illness is quite different from that of trigeminal neuralgia. It is much duller and more persistent, lasting hours rather than seconds and is not associated with the trigger factors of classical *tic doloureux*. It is not relieved by analgesics. The chest pain most typical of this condition is left submammary, radiating towards the axilla. It is not associated with exercise or position. It may come on at any time and it too is not relieved by analgesics.

Having decided that the greater part of the symptoms are due to anxiety, the doctor has to tell the patient that this is what he thinks. He should do this before he starts asking her about possible areas of stress in her life. She should be allowed to decide for herself whether she wants his help in dealing with her anxiety and any precipitating causes. She may have come to the doctor to find out whether she was suffering from organic disease needing treatment. Once she has the answer to this question, she may decide to deal with the problem herself or seek help from any of a number of other agencies. To write out a prescription for valium as soon as the diagnosis is made is to suggest that she is incapable of any action on her own behalf. If she does ask him to help her, then he clearly has to explain the different ways of proceeding open to her. One of these might be to take tranquillisers, another might be to see a community psychiatric nurse and try to sort out any problems. If she is aware of the source of her difficulties then the best method may be obvious. She may need help to get her difficult three-year-old into a nursery school, treatment for her alcoholic husband, the intervention of a social worker to stop the electricity supply from being cut off or find a place for grandmother in an old people's home.

As in depression, the main purpose of treatment is to help the woman to develop insight into her reactions and to improve her situation. Drugs play a negligible part in this process. In particular tranquillisers and hypnotics are best avoided. However, if after hearing the pros and cons from the doctor, the patient decides she would like to use them, most doctors would not refuse a small supply. Great care must be taken to see that the patient does not collect repeat prescriptions for ever after. Sometimes a β-blocker will help some of the symptoms of anxiety. Most of those now available seem safe and free from side-effects as long as they are not given to anyone with a history of heart failure or bronchospasm and a watch is kept for bradycardia and hypotension.

Women suffering from anxiety states are likely to have anxious personalities and will return again and again to the doctor with further symptoms. Many can be enabled to understand their own problems and how to handle them. They develop a high degree of insight and approach the doctor apologetically with a wry smile asking only for a few words of reassurance and comfort. If the doctor can avoid being impatient and patronising he can, with the rest of the team, help them to lead normal lives.

Note

1. G.W. Brown and T. Harris, *Social Origins of Depression* (Tavistock Publications, London, 1978).

12 WOMEN ALONE AND HANDICAPPED WOMEN

Women Alone

The traditional virgin spinster, left on the shelf because of a shortage of men, may belong to a previous age, but there is an increasing number of women who are not married or living in long-term relationships, either through choice or force of circumstances. They are not a homogeneous group. Some are alone because they are unable to form close, lasting relationships. Others have had such relationships which have broken down. Some of those desirous and capable of sharing their lives nevertheless lack the initiative and degree of extroversion needed to go out and meet people and make new friends from among whom they might find partners. Some have never married, some are widows or divorcees, some have children who may be with them or elsewhere. They all have different and quite individual problems and some, who are well adjusted and happy with their lot, have very few. Life for women on their own can be exciting and fulfilling, but there are pitfalls and some of the difficulties are common to all of them. They may not be any more numerous than those facing married women but they are as difficult to avoid and to handle. The main problem areas are housing, finance, social intercourse and emotional fulfilment. These are all to some extent linked. Women are traditionally poorly paid and recent legislation has made little impact on this so far. It is therefore difficult for them to buy or rent accommodation on the private market. They have low priority on council housing lists and may have to wait years for a council house or flat. In the meantime they have to live with parents or in lodgings. Both of these make normal social life difficult. They may have only a bedroom which is their own and cannot ask friends in for a cup of tea or a meal. Social intercourse therefore takes place in public, which is stultifying and expensive.

If a single woman lives with her parents for a long time, while waiting for accommodation of her own, they may be aged and dependent on her by the time she is able to leave. Even if they are not, they may find it difficult to understand why she wants to go and be hurt by her decision. If she has stayed so long partly because she found it hard to break the emotional ties and stand on her own feet, then the extra difficulties of establishing her own independent social and emotional life, while living with her parents, may make it impossible for her ever to leave. She may then feel trapped and resentful. Attempts at living away from her parents produce intense anxiety and she has to return, perhaps with an excuse to cover the real reason. This is a situation where the counsellor has to be particularly aware of the woman's limited scope for action. It may be obvious, and she herself may be able to see, that it would be best for her to live apart from her parents but if she is unable to make the break then this line of action is closed to her, at least at present. She may need skilled psychotherapy to overcome her difficulties. Like any other woman under stress, she is likely to have a low health quotient and may present to the doctor with apparently unrelated symptoms of organic or neurotic illness. Even if he is not willing or able to help her himself, he should be watching for underlying problems so that he can refer her to an appropriate colleague.

Emotional fulfilment and sexual satisfaction are often difficult for single women to achieve. This sometimes leads to an excessive dependence on relationships at work and intense distress over apparently minor disturbances. Many people have lively fantasies, which are usually harmless and may even be beneficial, but if they become intense or form a major part of life, then they can be destructive. If a woman has elaborate fantasies about people with whom she works, she may be abnormally sensitive to their behaviour and unable to relate to them normally. To lead a satisfactory life and maintain a balanced attitude to her work and her colleagues, she has to make a special effort to cultivate her leisure and social and intellectual interests away from her job. In most areas, there are many opportunities for this but some women may need help and support in order to take advantage of them. The very reason that such a woman finds herself alone and socially isolated is that relationships are difficult for her. She may be quite unable to join a club or evening class on her own, facing strangers on strange ground. Group psychotherapy may be helpful or the church may be able to draw her into its activities little by little. She might agree to help on a school or old people's outing, where she will feel safe, and gradually join other activities. Her only entrée into social life may be through her contact with the members of the primary health care team, who are the only people in a position to appreciate her difficulties and recognise her needs.

Sexual problems are particularly difficult to approach in a single woman. She is unlikely to complain of her frustration or anxiety directly and is more likely to come because of general malaise or pelvic discomfort or neurotic symptoms. She may not admit, even to herself, that her complaints are related to sexual anxiety or dissatisfaction. Even if she does, then it may seem that little can be done to put matters right.

However, if she can be enabled to discuss the problems, it may be possible to allay her anxiety, to reassure her that masturbation and sexual fantasies are not wicked or dangerous unless she thinks they are. Her sex life may still be imperfect but perhaps she will be able to live with it more comfortably.

As she approaches middle age she will have similar anxieties to everyone else. Anything she has not yet achieved and is not in sight of, she will be unlikely to achieve now. If she always longed to have a husband, children or a stable home with someone she loved and has not found them by the time she is forty, she probably never will.

On the other hand, if she is happy and well adjusted, she should still have time and energy to continue full-time work and gain promotion if she wants it, expand and develop her interests and relationships outside work and to lead an even more satisfying life than in the past. If she has not managed to solve the problems of loneliness, social isolation and emotional disability then her difficulties will increase as she grows older. She can no longer realistically hope and expect to make a better job of life in the future. Any plans she makes will have a hollow ring if they depend on her making social or emotional adjustments of which she is incapable. Her health quotient will not naturally increase with age and if she is unhappy then it will deteriorate.

She should be given every encouragement to make the most of her assets and expand her interests, but the counsellor should not expect too much of her. Any help she receives will probably be more in the nature of support than an attempt at change.

Homosexual women have similar social problems to homosexual men but often in a more acute form. Society views them with greater distaste and considers them more unnatural than their male counterparts. Some are swept into marriage when very young before fully understanding their sexual orientation and without realising how distasteful heterosexual marriage would be to them. Many are able to establish happy, stable, long-term relationships and develop a circle of friends who accept them completely. A few seem to exacerbate the problems of social acceptability by making their homosexuality into a way of life which is incomprehensible to even their most enlightened and sympathetic friends, whose own sexuality is more subdued or for the most part confined to private situations. Every activity, from work to sport, music-making or card games, proclaim their sexual orientation and this sets them apart in a way in which the mere fact of being homosexual would not. This social aggression seems to spring from fear and insecurity and makes them demanding and very difficult to help.

Women Alone and Handicapped Women

As with every other woman, the ability of a lesbian to cope with her problems depends on her background, upbringing, maturity and stability of personality. When these fail her, she may need help from members of the primary health care team even more than the heterosexual woman because of her difficulty in confiding in other people in the community. Doctors have to be particularly aware of physical symptoms which may be a smokescreen obscuring more important emotional difficulties. It is more than ever necessary for the counsellor to be blatantly unshockable and hide his own prejudices or feelings of distaste, if he is to enable a homosexual woman to talk about her problems and thereby help her to deal with them.

Widows and divorced women have to learn to live alone after a period of family life and home-making and in many ways this is more difficult than the life of the woman who never marries. The emotional stresses of bereavement and bitterness may affect the divorcee, who grieves for her marriage as well as railing against her husband, as much as the widow, who is resentful of her loneliness as well as grieving for her husband. If she married young and the marriage lasted a long time it is likely to be particularly difficult for her to find a job when in middle life she becomes dependent on work both financially and for company. She may lack both the information as to how to find suitable work or training and the drive to set about it. The primary health care team is in an ideal position, first to recognise her need, which she may not do herself, and secondly to help her to satisfy it.

One-parent Families

One of the results of the modern nuclear family is that if the marriage breaks down and the partners separate, the woman is usually left to bring up the children alone with little or no support from adult relations. As we have seen in Chapter 8, raising children is a complex task fraught with difficulties even when both parents are working together in harmony. Few couples can ever claim to have achieved complete success in it. For a single parent, whether unmarried, widow or divorcee, the difficulties are greatly magnified.

There is nearly always a severe and chronic shortage of money. If she goes out to work, she is unlikely to earn enough to support her family, and the more she earns, the less help she will receive from other sources. If she stays at home to care for her children, she may have little opportunity for adult company. If she is ill, she has to find someone to meet the children from school and care for them at home. She has to find a babysitter to cover every activity outside the home, from visiting the school for a parents' evening to going to the dentist or having her hair done. Her social life is severely limited. Most of her contemporaries will be married and she is likely to have lost touch with the friends she had before she married. A single woman is not as socially acceptable as a married couple and will not receive the same invitations from friends and neighbours. It is difficult for her to entertain herself. Even if she joins a club or evening class, she has to find and pay a babysitter and organise her own transport. Introducing a male friend into the family may be difficult.

The practical problems are therefore immense, but it is the emotional ones which cause the greatest strain and which have the most serious and damaging long-term effects on the children.

It is only by having a satisfying and stable emotional life herself that a woman can keep the problems of motherhood in perspective and maintain sensible and unstressful relationships with her children. Unless she is exceptionally mature and emotionally independent and stable, a single woman is unlikely to be able to provide her children with the calm, confident, consistent, parental love and support they need. In the absence of sources and objects of adult affection for herself she will depend too heavily on her children for her own emotional needs, which they cannot possibly satisfy. Minor problems become disproportionately important when there is no one to discuss them with, the standards of behaviour she sets for the children may be unattainably high and her tolerance of their inevitable failure limited.

Few women are able to hide their feelings of resentment towards the children's father, and the children are torn between love for him and feelings of guilt that, in continuing to love him, they are betraying her. They are angry with him for going and also feel in some way to blame. 'If I had been better he would have loved me more. If he had loved me more, he would not have left me.' Most of these powerful emotions are unconscious and result in a confused child with a reduced health quotient. He may develop neurotic symptoms, underachieve at school, or indulge in angry, aggressive antisocial behaviour such as vandalism or fighting.

His mother is already having difficulty coping with her own practical and emotional problems. Her own health quotient is low. She cannot handle her unhappy child.

The members of the primary health care team are likely to know of the breakdown of the marriage at an early stage and are in an ideal position to prepare the woman for the problems that she is going to face and work with her to prevent their worst results. A psychiatric nurse or social worker may be able to help the truncated family to work through its difficulties before they have caused lasting damage and irretrievable breakdown in relationships. Sometimes a court welfare officer, usually a probation officer, is involved and may be a great help. Links between this person and the primary health care team are very useful.

A woman bringing up a family on her own may need help in a number of areas such as housing, finance, work, child-minding and nursery schools, but it is her emotional and social problems which are most important. She needs to learn how to maintain her self-respect, build a life for herself as an individual as well as being a mother and member of a family, achieve a reasonable social life and emotional, intellectual and sexual fulfilment, and be a loving, consistent and supportive parent without becoming overdependent on her children. She needs to come to terms with the failure of her marriage and her own part in it and to deal with her feelings of anger and resentment towards her husband. She has to facilitate a continuing and loving relationship between him and the children. The children also need help in accepting the changed situation and in learning to understand and cope with their own sometimes violent emotions. It may be impossible for their mother to give them this help and a skilled and experienced health team worker is invaluable.

If help from the primary health care team is not forthcoming, the health of this mother and her children may well deteriorate. In time she will become an unhappy and unhealthy old woman and her children will be the next generation of unhappy, unhealthy parents unable to form and sustain mature relationships and lasting marriage, raising yet another generation with a low health quotient.

The central position of the primary health care team, the scope of its preventive work and the importance of its links with other agencies such as schools, police (juvenile bureau), probation officers and churches are clearly demonstrated by this situation.

Step-parents

One of the best things that can happen to a single woman with children is for her to marry. Much of the pressure on her as a single parent is relieved if she can share her problems with her husband and achieve emotional fulfilment through her relationship with him, lessening her dependence on the children. However, it is never easy to step into a ready-made family and take up a position previously occupied by someone else. Similar problems face a woman as a stepmother as face a man in his role as stepfather. Some of the problems are obvious and easily anticipated. The step-parent is compared, often unfavourably, to his or her predecessor. Firmness and discipline are resented by the children on the grounds that 'he is not our real father'. Affection and attempts at friendship are often viewed with suspicion. As well as these, there are less obvious emotional difficulties for children in adjusting to a step-parent. They may feel jealous of their mother's attachment to their stepfather and resent the amount of her time and attention he occupies. They may feel that to accept him and to love him would represent a betrayal of their own father. They may fear that this marriage too will fail and that one or other parent may leave them abandoned for a second time.

A child in this position sometimes builds up a defence system which prevents him from loving anyone in an attempt to protect himself from getting hurt. He then suffers chronic and continuing hurt and emotional deprivation which may show itself in a number of different ways: illness, either physical or psychiatric, neurotic symptoms, withdrawal, delinquency. More than anything, he needs parental love. Both parents are prepared to give it to him but he cannot allow them to. The members of the primary health care team know about this family. If they are aware of the problems that often arise for step-parents and children, they can make themselves available to help at an early stage and prevent irrevocable harm to the family.

Childless Couples

There have always been a proportion of couples who would have been better not to have children. Some lack the emotional resources to cope with a family, some have absorbing careers, others dislike children or have a deep-rooted difficulty in accepting them. It is therefore refreshing to find that in modern society more and more couples feel free to choose not to have children. There are still social pressures on them to conform to the accepted norm but they are not now nearly so strong and more reliable contraception makes the whole situation much easier for them. Young couples, childless by choice, may have little contact with the primary health care team except relating to contraception. This may present problems if they request sterilisation. Most doctors would be reluctant to support this if either of them is under thirty, however strongly they feel about it, but it may be difficult to explain this reluctance to the couple's satisfaction. It is of course based on the knowledge that people change as they mature and may feel differently in a few years' time. Also, the marriage may break down and each may have a change of heart with a new partner. The doctor can only do his best and try to help them find satisfactory contraception until it is clear that they have a stable marriage and views which are unlikely to alter further.

The team will have far more contact with those childless couples who want to have children and cannot. Initially they come for advice, investigation and referral and later for comfort or treatment of the results of the unhappiness and reduced health quotient caused by their infertility. Many couples find it very difficult to accept. Some women feel that their whole purpose in life has been destroyed. If the cause of the infertility is pinned on to one or other of the partners, there are the stresses of shame, guilt, blame and resentment to be dealt with within the marriage. They may want to consider adoption or AID with all their attendant difficulties and emotional connotations. After everything else has been considered, they have to be helped to make the most of their lives without children. This is sometimes frustrating work for the counsellor when the couple seem obstinately to refuse to see what advantages they have in the way of physical fitness, financial security and freedom to do as they please, and do nothing but bewail their lack of children. As with the grief of bereavement, it seems that this is a phase some people have to live through. All the counsellor can do is to provide comfort and support until it passes.

Handicapped Women

Women can be handicapped by physical or psychiatric disease, mental deficiency, emotional disability or by more than one of these. The difficulties which arise from physical and mental handicap depend a great deal on factors other than the disabling condition itself. The family circumstances, financial position, housing and extent of community support and facilities available all influence the precise nature of the difficulties. The most important factor is the woman's own underlying personality and emotional stability. A blind woman with a strong personality and emotional resources may have a high health quotient and few problems, and those she has she can handle herself with little assistance. Another, without these qualities, may be defeated by her handicap and need constant help and support. The majority lie between these extremes and can be enabled to lead healthy, satisfying, independent lives if they receive the right help when it is most needed.

Physical handicap of all sorts makes it difficult for a woman to lead a normal social life, to work and run a home. Mobility, transport, finance and housing are all matters about which she may need advice.

The members of the primary health care team should have information about how to obtain financial and practical help, for instance with special equipment, aids and alterations to the home. She may need help and support from a health worker to learn to adjust to and accept her disability and make the most of her positive qualities. Involvement with other members of the community is important and can often be initiated by a member of the primary health care team. If her appearance is abnormal, it may be particularly difficult for her to go out and meet people on her own. The church or care group may help her to become integrated into the community.

Psychiatric illness and mental handicap present especially difficult problems for families and the community and it is often with these, as much as with the handicapped individual, that the primary health care team must work. Sometimes quite simple intervention of a very basic kind can forestall disaster. Recently a mentally handicapped girl, who had previously been cared for by her mother, became estranged from her family when her parents' marriage broke down. She had a job in a local factory and married a man also suffering from mental deficiency, who also worked there. Neither of them could cook or shop or knew how to obtain accommodation. A distant relative offered them lodgings at an exorbitant rent and a long way from their work. They began to get behind with the rent and were in danger of losing their jobs because of constant lateness, undernourishment and exhaustion. A word from a member of the primary health care team to the local authority housing department obtained an immediate response and a flat. Contact was re-established with the girl's mother and resulted in lessons in basic shopping and cooking, and an ingenious scheme with a calendar and a pencil established the girl on the contraceptive pill. This couple are now self-sufficient, happy and healthy.

Many schizophrenic women can lead normal lives for long periods if their medication is administered regularly and the dosage adjusted carefully. This supervision is ideally provided by a community psychiatric nurse, working as a member of a primary health care team. She can also provide support, when necessary, for other members of the family and work closely with other members of the team such as the health visitor, who may be involved if there are young children in the family. The future of the whole family depends on the success of the teamwork in this situation.

The emotionally disabled form the largest group of handicapped people in the community and their problems are among the most complex and difficult to resolve. They are often not recognised but the effects of their handicap are far-reaching and disastrous. They include marital breakdown, alcoholism, attempted suicide, emotional deprivation and delinquency in children. A woman who is an emotional cripple is likely to have a low health quotient and therefore to be well known to the primary health care team. If the team is working well and on the look-out for this problem, she should be recognised without great difficulty. Appropriate help will not alter her basic personality but she may be enabled to live more satisfactorily within her own limitations and to learn how to protect her family from the worst effects of her disability. She and her husband may be able to develop enough insight into and understanding of her difficulties to enable the marriage to continue and the family to thrive.

The children of a handicapped woman may need special help. If she is confined to the house, they may need to be taken to and from school, to see the doctor or dentist, to buy clothes. There may be members of the family who can help with these matters, but if not the primary health care team can often act as a link between the family and a neighbour or education department or voluntary organisation. More difficult to handle are the problems which arise for the children in accepting their mother's disability and explaining it to their peers. This is an especially difficult problem if she looks abnormal when other children can be very unkind and make her own children ashamed of her.

Women with Handicapped Children

Women with handicapped children are all known to someone in the primary health care team, and although many of them need long-term help their problems are long-standing and not usually acute and they are therefore particularly easy to forget. Special attention needs to be given to ways of keeping them under regular review so that they are not neglected. There is always a flurry of concern and activity when a handicap is first recognised but the family may be lost sight of during the years that follow.

Despite the initial concern, the mother's problems are not always lessened by the quality of help she receives during the early stages. It is essential that both parents are fully informed by someone as senior as possible at all stages once anxiety about a child has been expressed. It is amazing how often people in a maternity ward fuss around a baby without explaining to the mother what is going on. She is left to ask whoever she can get hold of — perhaps the ward maid or a new pupil midwife. A general practitioner may refer a baby to a paediatrician by saying to the mother: 'I would like Dr Smith to have a look at John.'

She may not dare ask why. The waves of panic induced by the uncertainty are far worse than any reaction to factual information. This does not mean that every mother has to be told in detail all the possible implications of what might be, but probably is not, wrong with her baby, but she should be kept in the picture. She is more in the position of a partner to the clinician in this situation than in almost any other and should be respected as such.

The emotional shock to a mother of discovering that her baby may not be completely normal is shattering. She is subject to a confused mixture of torments: fear about the extent and effect of the abnormality, guilt at being responsible for it, anxiety that she will not be able to love the child enough to compensate him, shame, embarrassment and resentment at not being able to be proud of him, grief for the normal child she has been deprived of. The woman will need help to handle all these emotions but it is no part of the counsellor's job to deny them. As with the grief of bereavement, they must be experienced and lived through. At the same time, a certain amount of concentration on the immediate practical issues and plans can be helpful. It is never too early to start emphasising the child's positive attributes. However awful his disability, he must have some endearing qualities, some potential for progress. He is likely to make the most of this potential if it is sought out and emphasised by his parents. They may need help and guidance to do this.

One of the worst aspects of having a handicapped child is the feeling of isolation, that no one else is in a similar position. It is a great help to the mother to be introduced to another woman with a similar problem or to join a club or group of parents who can share their experience, expertise and ingenuity, which is often impressive. They may then also be able to develop a feeling of hope and enthusiasm which is difficult to sustain if the family's only social contacts are friends and neighbours with normal children. The members of the primary health care team should be able to effect such introductions or even start a club themselves, if there is not one already in the area.

Just as every human being is unique and has problems like no one else's, so every handicapped child is special and different from every other. The difficulties he and his family experience will be different from those even of other people with the same handicapping condition. It is not possible to say that all mongols or all spastic children have a particular problem, and it is dangerous and unhelpful to lump them all together. However, there are areas of difficulty shared by all families with handicapped children. They include financial problems, education, mobility, babysitting, the slower rate of progress of the child in some areas, social adjustments and holidays. All these are matters that are within the scope of the primary health care team to help by providing information, ideas, introductions, encouragement and support. The terrible isolation of the family can thereby be lessened and the inevitable episodes of despair reduced.

It is important that, in caring for the handicapped child to the best of her ability, the mother does not neglect her own interests, her marriage and her other children. It would not benefit him if she did. He needs a happy, secure, loving family as much as anyone. His ability to deal with his difficulties in the future depend upon it. The quality of his upbringing depends not so much on devoted self-sacrifice on the part of his mother but on her building a happy family for him. This necessitates maintaining her own self-respect, individuality and personal interests in the same way as any other woman. She may need much encouragement to do this when the burden of duty seems always to be calling on her to service the needs of her extradependent child. It is important for him to be treated as normally as possible and this means that everyone around him must learn to behave normally. As the handicapped child grows, the mother may be faced with the prospect of having to care for him forever. Every effort should be made to integrate him as far as possible into the community in a sheltered workshop, adult training centre or even residential home so that the burden on the parents does not become intolerable and his future is safeguarded in case there comes a time when they are no longer able to care for him.

Throughout the life of a handicapped individual, his family and especially his mother are subjected to stress of a particularly wearing kind. They may need a great deal of help if this is not to lower their health quotient.

13 TEAM SUPPORT FOR A WOMAN'S HEALTH

It is clear that a woman's health is founded on many factors, some inborn, some environmental, some physical, some emotional, some social, some domestic, some arising from her background and upbringing, some from her present situation. Many of these factors are unalterable. They cannot be influenced by anything either the woman herself or the members of the primary health care team can do. However, the level at which she functions, her degree of health and happiness, her quality of life, may be affected by quite small changes. The timely provision of appropriate help and care can enable her to cope in adverse circumstances and to overcome some of the difficulties with which she is surrounded. She may then be able to raise herself and her family to a higher level of health.

The diverse nature of the problems which may affect a woman's health mean that a team approach is needed if appropriate help is to be available. It cannot be provided by any one individual, however experienced, well trained and enthusiastic, nor can it be provided satisfactorily by a group of different individuals working separately. A woman and her problems cannot be divided up into compartments, each being helped by a different person. She must function as an integrated whole and any help she receives needs to be closely co-ordinated.

Primary care is not at present organised in such a way as to provide co-ordinated help and care. The changes needed will be examined in this chapter.

The Concept of Health

The training of most of the people who come together to form a primary health care team is based on the central concept of illness, its diagnosis and treatment. Most of them see illness as a positive entity with a clear cause, health is the absence of illness and not the other way round. If our understanding of women's health is to improve, it must be viewed as a positive attribute, which may sometimes be lost, threatened, interrupted or diminished. Illness is something which may then intervene. Such an about-turn will be extremely difficult for most people. Some may even find it threatening. If your work is centred on the diagnosis and treatment of illness, illness then becomes the whole point of your work. To have it demoted to second place in importance to an apparently nebulous concept called health, seems to detract from the value of what you do. However, to emphasise the superiority of the concept of health over that of disease is not to belittle the work of caring for the sick and diagnosing and treating disease. This must be done but it must be done in the context of re-establishing health and not as an end in itself.

If we can only undo some of the inhibiting effects of our training, we should not find it difficult to accept health as a positive attribute and learn to understand it. Anyone can recognise health, or its absence, in a friend or relative. There is a bloom, a radiance, in a healthy person, regardless of age or sex, which is immediately recognisable. It shows in his skin colour and texture, his muscle tone, his bright eyes and voice, the way he holds his head and hands, the way he moves. All this is lost in the unhealthy. The slack, flat look, the dull eyes and skin, the limp muscles, drooping spine are immediately obvious. If everyone else can recognise this, then surely the professional health worker can allow himself to do so too.

The Role of the Primary Health Care Team

It is easy to speculate, even romanticise, about what primary health care teams might in theory attempt to do. It is much more difficult, some might say impossible, to put the theory into practice. I do not underestimate the difficulties but I do claim that this work is not only what we should all be attempting to do: that the end is itself both possible and desirable and that it is a proper way to conduct primary care, but also that everyone would benefit from making the attempt.

My thesis is based on the belief that the future of health care lies in people working together. It is one of the few fields where there is universality of interest. Every member of society is involved, whether he is employed in health care or not. If the health quotient of the population is to be raised, people will have to work together — within individual relationships, within families, community organisations, primary health care teams and hospitals. If this happened, the needs of the sick and handicapped would be better served and it might also be possible to improve the health of the community. At the same time, there is little doubt that the quality of life for those working in health care would be improved. There would be fewer frustrations, less strain and a greater degree of personal fulfilment.

The Need for Change

However, this is not the way the health service works at present and major changes would be needed for it to happen: changes in the attitudes of people to their work and to each other, changes in methods of working, changes in the content of the work and, perhaps most important, changes in the attitude of the community towards health and sickness.

At present, health care is carried out by individuals working alone and coming together only occasionally and for the most part informally. When groups meet to discuss ideas or formulate policy, it is usually within their own discipline. Nurses meet to discuss the latest techniques and share problems they have in working with doctors and administrators; receptionists meet to pool their experiences and share the problems they have in working with nurses and doctors and administrators; doctors meet to try to keep up to date, sharpen their wits against each other and share the problems they have with patients and nurses and administrators. Such meetings may be useful but they also serve to exaggerate the separateness of the members of the team and make it more difficult for them to work together.

In primary health care, even where the rudiments of a team exist in terms of personnel and premises, the work is usually still being done in separate compartments. The health visitor may have an office in the central practice premises but she is doing the same work as she always did and may have little contact with anyone else in the building. She visits the babies, of whose birth she is notified through official channels, and organises a baby clinic and help for old people, when it is needed, but she may work in almost total isolation from other members of the team. The district nurse and midwife may be 'attached' to the practice but this does not mean that they meet anyone else working in the same practice or even enter the building any more often than they previously did. They receive messages or instructions from the doctor. They do not necessarily work with him. The team exists only in theory. It does not work as a team but as a group of separate individuals with a common base. The lines of demarcation are clear and often rigidly adhered to, the hierarchy is well established.

In most instances, the establishment of a primary health care team happens gradually over a long period. It is not planned and the members do not come together specifically to work as a team. Each brings with him his own idea of his job. It is the same job as he has been doing already, or has been trained to do, and it does not include the concept of working closely with others except over particular situations as they arise. There is no room for close liaison and planning, no room for sharing problems and decision-making, for resolving difficulties. Not only is this wasteful and inefficient but it results in tremendous strain on the individuals concerned, each working in relative isolation. The strain affects all members of the team, and sometimes even the patients, but it is greatest for the doctors. Their tradition of personally carrying the whole burden of responsibility for the organisation of the practice, as well as the clinical care of each patient, is well established and regarded by most as unalterable. Few feel able to share the burden even with each other. Even within a group practice, each doctor usually works alone, keeping his anxieties about clinical problems, his irritation with his colleagues, his frustrations and his often immense emotional exhaustion, to himself. It does none of them any good and, for some, the strain is intolerable. The incidence of marital breakdown, alcoholism and suicide in doctors is among the highest for any group.

The Fear of Change

The system continues because it is upheld by tradition and because few people can envisage any workable alternative. It is generally accepted to be part of the doctor's job to carry heavy responsibility and no one questions whether all of it is necessary or desirable. To share his burden might be to dilute his worth, both in his own eyes and in those of society as a whole. He may not be able to see how limited is his scope when he works in isolation, that his expertise might be better used and on a broader front, that to work within a team could increase his value.

Other members of the team have similar problems. For them too it is easier to continue an established pattern of work than to step out into the unknown.

True teamwork inevitably involves an element of audit. This is one of its advantages. A critical examination has to be made of the work of each member, both by himself and by the rest of the team, as well as an examination of the work of the team as a whole. As a result, everyone's work may be modified: some tasks will be shared, some reallocated, some changed, some deemed unnecessary and jettisoned. The idea of such events is threatening and frightening as well as exciting. It is difficult to appreciate what the advantages of working as a member of a team might be before they are experienced. The overriding feeling is fear of change. It is therefore not surprising that the establishment of working primary health care teams has been slow and patchy and that pressure to change does not always come from within the team.

A further problem arises from the established attitudes and expectations of the general public. Most people are frightened by symptoms of illness, however benign, and are not prepared to take responsibility for themselves and their families in matters of sickness or health. In most areas, the general practitioner is the only professional health worker to whom they feel they can turn and they have come to expect him to be always available and to provide immediate treatment whether or not it is appropriate to their ailment. It is a slow process to replace the general practitioner by a team, of which he is just one member, and to teach the public to make proper use of such a team.

However, it is possible to effect change and some movement is already beginning. It is not difficult now to envisage a gradual evolution towards a different sort of health service based on teamwork and co-operation. The process is starting at the level of primary care.

How to Start

It is theoretically possible to imagine a situation, for instance in a new town or housing estate, where a practice could be set up where no health care facilities had previously existed and where all the members of the team could be appointed to posts which are advertised as being based on teamwork. In this situation, everyone joining the practice would do so knowing that his work was going to be, in many ways, different from anything he had done before and would bring with him flexibility of outlook and enthusiasm for the task. The local population would have no preconceived ideas about what to expect from this new practice and would therefore be more likely to accept something unusual.

For most people interested in establishing a primary health care team, the reality is very different. Most of the personnel already work in the practice. Many of them have never considered alternative ways of working and may be hostile to new ideas. Change has to be introduced gradually and on a very limited scale. The initiative can come from anyone working in the practice. It should not be too difficult to persuade a few members of the team to meet together to discuss a specific problem, perhaps an individual patient or the organisation of appointments or repeat prescriptions. If the meeting is pleasant and fruitful, further meetings may be arranged, perhaps on a regular basis. Attendance would have to be voluntary and some members may never come. Gradually some of these occasions may include most of the team and there may be opportunities to discuss broad ideas and general principles. The pattern of meetings will depend on the perceived needs of the members. Many will be small and informal involving only a few people, others may include everyone and have to be more formal. Some may include people from outside the team, invited for a particular discussion.

The doctors are likely to find it most difficult to join interdisciplinary discussions in a relaxed way. They feel constantly under pressure and may look upon meetings as a waste of valuable time. Some may tend to take over the meeting and make it difficult for other members to express themselves. In the early stages of the development of the team, those members who feel themselves low in the scale of importance may hesitate to say anything at all when the doctors are there. It can be a help if some very small meetings are held to discuss aspects of the work which directly involve such people so that they can get used to speaking out.

A doctor may hesitate to discuss a patient's problems in a practice meeting because of anxiety about confidentiality. However, he will gradually come to realise that patients often tell the receptionist more about the details of their private lives than they tell the doctor and that confidentiality is something which can be respected by all members of the team.

The fact that meetings are taking place at all very soon reduces tensions within the practice and relationships flourish. Several members of the team are likely to have problems with the same patient and will share their anxieties and rationalise care, so that overlap lessens and contradictory advice is eliminated. Enthusiasm for working together gradually increases. As time goes by, the team will develop a broad common philosophy, or basis, for its work which might be expressed in terms of long-term objectives reached by means of short-term aims.

The following headings might be included:

Objectives (Long-term)

1. A comprehensive and effective service for the care of the sick and dying.
2. A higher health quotient for the members of the community.
3. Greater self-sufficiency in the community in relation to health and sickness.
4. Greater integration into community life of the handicapped and disabled.

Aims (Short-term)

To work together as a team
– to provide an advisory and treatment service for the management of acute and chronic sickness, linking closely with the hospital service and with agencies in the community and involving the patient and his family as partners in the process
– to prevent ill health by identifying vulnerable people and those at risk or suffering from disease at an early stage; helping individuals and families to improve their health quotient; providing screening and

immunisation programmes where appropriate
— to educate the public in matters of health and sickness and the use of services
— to safeguard the confidentiality of information about patients
— to identify and exploit the particular skills and interests of individual members of the team
— to examine regularly the work of the practice, critically and in detail, identify areas of friction, new needs, gaps in the service, opportunities for improvement, and make appropriate changes
— to develop systems of working together which are both efficient and flexible
— to examine new ideas to improve the service
— to help and support each other.

These aims will be easier to achieve if it can be accepted that many of the tasks performed by the primary health care team can be done by any one of several members and that even work which might best be done by one person may in fact have to be done by another or not at all, depending on factors other than the skills and training of the individual. An alcoholic woman whose children had recently been taken into care desperately needed help. She felt unable to talk to the doctors or social workers, who had been involved in the court case, but was able to relate to one receptionist who tided her over until she felt less bitter and was able to start to rebuild her life. The district nurse is often in a better position to choose the right dressing for a leg ulcer, or drug for a dying patient, than the doctor. The community psychiatric nurse may sometimes be more likely to make an accurate assessment of the risk of injury to a child in a family than the social worker.

This abolition of lines of demarcation is difficult for some people to accept but as long as it evolves gradually and any difficulties are shared, this need not be a bar to progress. In fact members of different disciplines can learn a great deal from each other if they are flexible enough and are prepared to do so. Gradually the equal-value principle, which is so important in families, in schools and within marriage, infiltrates the primary health care team and at this point, the full benefit of teamwork begins to be felt. The hierarchical system dissolves and the burden on the individual members lessens. An increase in goodwill is evident. The time the doctor spends in meetings is soon made up by the sharing of clinical care which becomes possible. Some of the routine visiting of old people is now done by the district nurse. The health visitor will see the woman with post-natal depression on some of the occasions, when she needs comfort and support. It should be possible to streamline the routine care of patients on long-term medication, such as diabetics, so that the receptionist checks when they are due to be seen and arranges appointments, the nurse carries out checks on weight, blood sugar and whatever other tests are due, and the doctor can limit himself to checking the results and perhaps briefly seeing the patient for any clinical examination which is necessary.

The Patients

The establishment of a working primary health care team is usually welcomed by the patients of the practice as long as it is presented to them as providing extra facilities and not as a way of making it more difficult for them to see the doctor. Full use of the team will take time to develop and will come about through several different channels. One of the commonest and most useful is through the receptionist. Patients will often mention anxieties to the receptionist and doubts about whether the doctor is the best person to see. Someone may come and say, 'I am worried about my mother. She lives alone and I really don't think she can manage.' The receptionist will say, 'Would you like to discuss it with the social worker?' and the link is established. A middle-aged woman may express anxiety about her daughter's marriage. The receptionist will tell her that the marriage guidance counsellor comes twice a week and would be happy to see the couple if they wanted to make an appointment. Similarly, the receptionist will let it be known that the nurse is the person to see in the first instance with cuts and grazes, warts and ear syringing. News of the facilities spreads by word of mouth and very soon people refer themselves to the member of the team most appropriate to their needs or whom they feel best able to approach. Sometimes this gives rise to anomalies such as the woman with a lump in the breast who first showed it to the nurse. The relaxed atmosphere in the practice enabled the nurse to ask the doctor to come in and see her there and then. She admitted she would never have found the courage to do anything about it in any other way.

A certain amount of more formally presented information is a good idea, particularly for people who are new to the practice. Probably one of the best innovations is a practice booklet containing basic facts about surgery opening hours, telephone numbers, names and designations of members of the team and details of how they may be contacted. It can go further and offer advice about how to use the services, how to make an appointment, when to call the doctor and a brief description of what each member of the team does. A further extension, or another leaflet, could deal with how to handle minor illnesses and accidents and medical emergencies. It could also contain a list of useful telephone numbers such as the local care group, social services department and Samaritans. Posters and a regular practice news sheet can also be useful sources of information for patients, but it must always be borne in mind that a sizable proportion of the population cannot read fluently and the written information cannot replace personal contact with the members of the team. This is what working together is all about.

Continuing to Grow

Every primary health care team will be different. No uniformity can be externally imposed. Each will develop its own identity. How it grows and changes will depend on local factors and on its members and the degree of democracy they establish. As new members are appointed, consideration should be given as to how they will fit in, what qualities they will bring and whether they are flexible enough to start a new job which will inevitably be different from their previous one.

Some teams will remain small in numbers and in diversity. Others will expand. The basic members are:

General Practitioner
Health Visitor
District Nurse
Midwife
Receptionist.

It is becoming more common for these to be added:

Community Psychiatric Nurse
Social Worker
Surgery Nurse
Nursing Auxiliary
Practice Manager
Chiropodist
Secretary
Marriage Guidance Counsellor.

There is no reason why in the future the team could not include:

Physiotherapist
Dietician
Teachers of yoga, meditation or keep-fit
Specialist family planning nurse
Nursery nurse to run a creche
Representatives from patients' organisation or local care group.

Once established, the team develops a momentum of its own, kept going by the drive and enthusiasm of its members. It is a tender plant needing constant attention but as long as it is not neglected or taken for granted, it will flourish and grow. It must never be allowed to become static or it will die. The old personal and professional jealousies will reappear, the acceptance of each member as of equal value will be lost, the aims of the team will become fragmented again, the sharing of work will stop and the common purpose will fade.

As long as this is not allowed to happen, as long as the members realise that the team is nothing without them and that it is up to each individual to play his part in keeping it going, it will thrive.

After a time it will develop stature and self-confidence and may be able to look outwards for ways to forge further links with other parts of the health service and other agencies. A future in which each community is served by an integrated health service where the health of women is of central importance is perhaps the greatest objective of all.

INDEX

abortion 68-9
adolescence 102; sexual development in 53-4
alcoholism 83, 149, 155
amenorrhoea 40-1; anorexia nervosa 40; depression 132; menopause 109; oral contraceptive 41; post-natal 41; puberty 40; Turner's syndrome 40
amniocentesis 72
anaemia 123
angina 123
anorexia nervosa 40
anxiety 25, 83, 97, 137-9; and depression 132

backache 107-8
battered babies 77, 79, 97
breast feeding 78, 94

carcinoma: of breast 107; of cervix 45, 107
cervical: polyps 45; smear 44
cervicitis 44
childbirth 70; fear of 73; place of 76
child guidance clinic 105
childless couples 146-7
children and marital problems 90-2
chiropodist 160
chiropody 122
chronic bronchitis 120
colic 78
conception 60-1
contraception 60-9, 81; cap 65-6; in middle age 113; intra-uterine device 66-7; oral 62-5; sheath 65
cot death 95

depression 83, 97, 129-37; and anxiety 138; in middle age 107-9; in old age 119; puerperal 77, 78, 81, 82, 133; treatment 133-7
developmental examinations 99
diabetes 124
dietitian 160
disability: emotional 111, 147-9; prevention 119-22

discipline 94
district nurse 10; and care of dying 127; and the team 154, 158, 160
divorced women 143
doctors 23, 26, 27-30; child care 94; depression 132; marriage counselling 84; post-natal care 79; sexual problems 48-52; teamwork 156-7, *see also* general practitioners
Down's syndrome 72
drugs: in depression 133-6; in elderly 124-6
dying, care of the 127
dysmenorrhoea 36-9
dyspareunia 43, 44, 110

emotional: development 101; disablement 111, 147-9; fulfilment 141; handicap 82; health in pregnancy 70, 72; independence 85-6, 101, 117-19; problems 103, 108; shock 150; stress 108; state in pregnancy 78
enuresis 100

family life 18, 20, 93-105
foetus 77, 78

general practitioner 10, 160; and handicapped children 149; and sexual problems 48, *see also* doctor
grief 128

handicapped children 149-51
handicapped women 147
headache: in depression 131; in middle age 107-8
health 10, 12; concept of 152-3; happiness 15-17, 23; foundations of 152; marriage 83; sexual problems 49
health quotient 12-13, 48, 96, 98, 151; and menstrual problems 36; in depression 130; in handicapped women 147; in middle age 106, 107, 108; in single women 141; of

Index

population 23, 153
health visitor 10; and handicapped women 148; and mothers 26-7, 32, 77, 82; and the team 154, 158, 160; and young families 79, 98, 99; work of 75
heart failure 123
home help 123
homosexual women 142-3
hormone replacement therapy 110-11
hospital admission. for elderly 123; in treatment of depression 136-7
hot flushes 110
hypertension 107, 119
hyperthyroidism 123
hysterectomy 107, 110

impotence 49
independence: emotional 85-6, 101, 117-19; in adolescence 101; in old age 116, 117
infertility 49, 60-1
ischaemic heart disease 119

keep-fit: class 120; teacher 160

leukoplakia 43, 45
libido 55-6; in depression 132
love: and sex 46; for new baby 74, 94; in marriage 84, 86

marital problems 49, 79, 83-92
marriage 83-92; breakdown in doctors 155; counselling 84; in old age 115; non-consummation 49, 50
marriage guidance counsellor 84, 88, 105, 111, 160
masturbation 49; in children 52-3; in old age 116
Mead, Margaret 18
medical records 30
meditation teacher 160
menopause 109-11
menorrhagia 36; in middle age 107
menstruation 35-45; dysmenorrhoea 36-9; normal cycle 35-6
middle age 106-13
midwife 10, 71, 77, 154, 160

nurse: family planning 160; nursery 160; surgery 160, *see also* district nurse, psychiatric nurse

nursing auxiliary 160

obedience: in adolescents 102, 105; in infants 94-7
obesity 119
old age 114-28
one-parent families 143-5
osteoarthritis 119
ovarian swellings 45

patients 27, 159
pelvic pain 44
physiotherapist 124, 160
post-coital bleeding 43, 45, 109
post-menopausal bleeding 43, 45
post-natal: care 78-82; depression 32, 82; examination 81
practice manager 160
pregnancy 70-6; blood pressure in 74; smoking in 71, 72; test 70; vomiting in 73
premature ejaculation 49, 56
premenstrual tension 41
primary health care team 10, 23, 25-34, 152-61; contraception 61; elderly 115, 119, 121-6; families 98, 103, 105; handicapped children 149; handicapped women 148; marriage counselling 83, 84, 87; one-parent families 144-5; pregnancy 77; post-natal care 80, 82; schools 33; sexual problems 48, 59; single women 141
psychiatric nurse 82, 84, 111; and the team 158, 160; depression 32, 134-7; one-parent families 144-5; schizophrenic women 148; sexual problems 57
puberty 101, *see also* adolescence
punishment 96-7, 103-4

questionnaire: for elderly 121-2; for patients 30-1

receptionist 26, 71, 81, 160
rheumatoid arthritis 107
rubella: in pregnancy 71; vaccination 61, 71

schizophrenic women 148
schools 33-4
Second World War 20
sex 46-59; after surgery 57-8; in old age 58-9, 116

sexual: behaviour 46; conditioning 46; development 53; identity 49; intercourse 47; problems 48-59, 141; roles 17, 47; technique 46; tensions 50
sexuality 46; in children 52
single women 140-3
sleeping problems 99-100
socialisation 19
social position of women 17
social worker 84, 111; and the team 158, 160; anxiety 138; depression 32, 134; elderly 124; one-parent families 145
speech therapy 122
step-parents 145-6
sterilisation 67-8
stress: birth 78; depression 132; infancy 80; family life 100, 103; marriage 83; middle age 107
stroke 119
suicide 83, 155

termination of pregnancy 68-9; following rubella 71
toilet training 95, 100
tranquillisers: in anxiety 138-9; in depression 133-4; in the menopause 110
trigeminal neuralgia 138
tubal ligation 68

urethral caruncle 43

vaginal: discharge 41-3; infections 44
vaginismus 49
varicose veins 107
vasectomy 67
venereal disease 43, 49
vulval warts 43

weaning 94
well-baby clinic 99
widow 114, 128, 140, 143

Yoga: class 120; teacher 160